Solving for Why

Solving For Why

**A Surgeon's Journey to
Discover the Transformative
Power of Purpose**

DR. MARK G. SHRIME

TWELVE

NEW YORK   BOSTON

Copyright © 2022 by Mark G. Shrime

Jacket design by Jarrod Taylor. Cover copyright © 2022 by Hachette Book Group, Inc.

Twelve
Hachette Book Group
1290 Avenue of the Americas, New York, NY 10104
twelvebooks.com
twitter.com/twelvebooks

First Edition: January 2022

Twelve is an imprint of Grand Central Publishing. The Twelve name and logo are trademarks of Hachette Book Group, Inc.

The publisher is not responsible for websites (or their content) that are not owned by the publisher.

The Hachette Speakers Bureau provides a wide range of authors for speaking events. To find out more, go to www.hachettespeakersbureau.com or call (866) 376-6591.

Library of Congress Cataloging-in-Publication Data

Names: Shrime, Mark, author.
Title: Solving for why : a surgeon's journey to discover the transformative power of purpose / Mark Shrime.
Description: First edition. | New York : Twelve, 2022. | Includes bibliographical references.
Identifiers: LCCN 2021033001 | ISBN 9781538734162 (hardcover) | ISBN 9781538734148 (ebook)
Subjects: LCSH: Shrime, Mark. | Surgeons—United States—Biography. | Traffic accident victims—United States—Biography. | Social medicine. | Self-realization.
Classification: LCC R154.S55 A3 2022 | DDC 617.092 [B]—dc23
LC record available at https://lccn.loc.gov/2021033001

ISBNs: 978-1-5387-3416-2 (hardcover), 978-1-5387-3414-8 (ebook)

Printed in the United States of America

LSC-C

Printing 1, 2021

To my parents, George and Souad:
I am proud to be your son

Contents

Introduction

I don't know Who—or what—put the question, I don't know when it was put. But at some moment I did answer Yes to Someone—or Something—and from that hour I was certain that existence is meaningful and that, therefore, my life, in self-surrender, had a goal.

—DAG HAMMARSKJÖLD

IF YOU CAN HELP it, don't get into a car accident in Liberia. It changes things.

This was 2008. Liberia was four and a half years out from a couple of back-to-back civil wars that cost nearly a million lives. Six years later, an Ebola epidemic would infect over ten thousand people and kill half of them.

The United Nations still maintained a strong presence in this small West African nation. Peacekeepers in light blue helmets patrolled the streets of its capital, Monrovia.

Fresh out of a surgical fellowship, I had been in the country for a few months, working as a cancer surgeon on a hospital ship, docked off the coast of Monrovia.

This particular weekend, twenty of us expats decided to take a trip three hours to the northwest, to Robertsport, a beach town close to the Sierra Leonean border. Robertsport is a mecca for surfers, the eastern Atlantic's waves hurling themselves against its sandy West African beach. The drive from Monrovia to Robertsport is simple. It requires one direction change: an hour north of Monrovia, you turn left.

The road out of the capital was paved; the road from the left-hand turn to Robertsport was unpaved, single-track, and made of packed red dirt—pretty flat, pretty well maintained, but punctuated by one-lane, rickety wooden bridges spanning shallow ravines.

The twenty of us arranged five taxis for the weekend. I'm using the word *taxi* a little generously here. Four years out from two civil wars, Liberia had yet to rebuild its infrastructure. These taxis were bright yellow cars, as you'd expect, but they didn't have fully contiguous floorboards. You could see the road running beneath your feet, a little like a *Flintstones* cartoon. And they were driven by people who couldn't have been more than twenty years old.

The thing with young men and cars is that we like to go fast. So, once our cars made that left-hand turn onto the red dirt road, the drivers took off. And we loved it. It was a weekend off work. The windows were down, the wind in our hair. We were away from the hospital ship, out of the city, and speeding deeper into the country.

We goaded the drivers on. The driver of my car was the fastest. He wove his way to the head of the pack. When he got there, he booked it, as fast as he could, on the straight parts of the road. Then, when he came to a bridge, he'd slow down and cross the bridge responsibly—and then book it again to the next bridge.

Here's the thing: if you barrel down a red dirt road and then suddenly stop, you kick up a bloom of dust behind you. The car behind us didn't see us. It rammed into us. We fell off the bridge and into the ravine.

They say that time slows down during an accident. And they're right.

I remember watching the ground approach the windshield. I remember thinking, *Huh. I guess this is how I die. And that's okay.*

The ground hit the windshield. The car was totaled. Thankfully none of us were totaled—we escaped with scrapes and bruises and a lot of whiplash. A contingent of UN peace-keepers from Pakistan happened to be driving down the road in the opposite direction. They saw the accident, pulled us out of the ravine, took us to their base, made sure we were all right, and bundled us into the remaining four taxis. We made it to Robertsport, had a fabulous weekend, and then drove back to Monrovia for work on Monday.

THERE'S BEEN A LOT of research on the time dilation that occurs in catastrophic and near-death experiences like car crashes. Valtteri Arstila, a Finnish researcher who studies the role of time in perceptions of experience, theorizes that this time dilation is due to a rapid ramping up of the normal cognitive processes that happen in our heads every day.[1] It's possible that this ramp-up is due to one of fourteen different neurotransmitters that are released right at the moment of death—including dopamine, a mediator of pleasure; glutamate, crucial for memory processing; and norepinephrine, which increases alertness.[2]

But there's another school of thought. Chess Stetson, Matthew

Fiesta, and David Eagleman—researchers at the California Institute of Technology, the University of Texas Medical School at Houston, and Baylor College of Medicine—took volunteers up a 150-foot-tall platform and asked them to fall backwards into a net. During their fall, the volunteers wore a wristwatch that flashed numbers too quickly for the normal mind to process.

Stetson and his colleagues theorized that if the brain actually ramped up its cognitive processes during terrifying experiences, then the volunteers would be able to read these faster-than-normal numbers during their fifteen-story fall. They couldn't, even though they still *felt* like time slowed down.[3]

The researchers concluded that time dilation is a subjective, *ex post facto* misremembering of the events that occur during a catastrophic or near-death experience.

Fascinating stuff.

But, to some degree, none of it matters to me. Because that thought—"This is how I die, and that's okay"—stayed with me for those two days in Robertsport, and has continued to stay with me for over a decade since.

I was at peace in 2008, because after fifteen years of working in a career I hated, I had solved for why. And with that had come wonder and faith and worship and meaning.

Stick with me. Let me tell you the story.

Chapter 1

He had not thought of himself as Other, as worthy of disapproval simply by virtue of being who he was. Well, of course, in reality, he was totally Other.

—SALMAN RUSHDIE

SINCE 2008, I'VE WORKED to bring surgical care to the world's forgotten poor. I've done it from the decks of hospital ships docked off coastal countries in sub-Saharan Africa, from within excrement-painted hospital walls in the highlands of Haiti, and from the self-important ivory towers of academia. Why?

Because I'm a surgeon who never wanted to be a doctor.

Because I'm an Arab who grew up thinking Arabs were dirty.

Because I work in Africa, but I used to pray I'd end up anywhere else.

Solving for why has been a tortuous path; its hairpin turns changed my life. I hope my story changes yours.

Before I can tell you the things I learned on that path, and before I can introduce you to my traveling companions—both the welcome ones like worship and faith and wonder, and the less-welcome ones like anxiety and failure and doubt—I need to tell you my story.

I need to tell you how a kid who hated medicine and who was taught to hold himself separate became a surgeon enmeshed in the dusty beauty of the Other. And I need to tell you about faith lost and worship regained. Let's get started.

I WAS A YEAR old the first time someone pointed a gun at me.

Backlit by a fierce Middle Eastern sun, he wore an ill-fitting, dirty uniform. Voices from the rabble of men he'd already forced out of their cars quieted. His vision narrowed to the six inches separating him, a one-year-old boy, and the boy's mother. He held the gun that connected them against her head.

Would he have to shoot this woman? Would he have to kill her baby? Or would the father finally step out of his car?

Behind the soldier stretched a long, bloody story, half a century of fathers murdered at their children's baptisms, of snipers and car bombs and barricades, of racism and nationalism, and of failing empires playing at geopolitics. A story of Othering. A story of setting ourselves apart. A story that was mine.

IT WOULDN'T BE THE last time someone pointed a gun at me. Thirty years later and seven thousand miles away, a man whose face I never saw pushed a double-barreled shotgun into my stomach. There was no fierce Middle Eastern sun that night. It was a moonless, late-autumn evening, the kind that folks in Texas live for.

The oppressive summer had begun to crack, letting in hints of the coming cool. Some houses had already lit their fireplaces; charred wood laced the air.

I had been at the hospital late that day, embroiled in the scut work of medical student life—unearthing patient charts, drawing blood, pushing beds, and scouring vending machines for anything that wasn't Cheez-Its. When I finally collapsed into my boxy, used Volvo, rolled the windows down, turned the music up, and started the forty-five-minute drive to my mom's house, I folded into a satisfied and tired calm.

In retrospect, I'd noticed the headlights behind me for at least ten minutes. My childhood home, where I lived for the first two years of medical school, sits in a nondescript residential neighborhood in Dallas, flanked by two-story strip malls, each anchored with unremarkable banks, grocery stores, and Tex-Mex restaurants. It's easy to get lost in the almost-parallel streets, among featureless lawns surrounding single, off-center oak trees.

The man wasn't lost. "Give me your money," he said.

It would have been cliché if it hadn't been so threatening. His voice was young, hesitating, reedy. His accent was distinctly non-American. He wasn't far out of puberty.

His shotgun didn't hesitate. He'd covered the stock with a towel. I could only see its twin barrels.

Would he have to shoot me? Or would I give up my money?

I pulled a confusion of receipts, credit cards, IDs, money, and keys from my pocket. Testament to his fear, he let me rifle through the jumble, picking out the cash and keeping the rest. Testament to my fear, I thought this was an excellent idea.

We stood in silence until he wised up, grabbed the entire wad, and drove off.

My computer sat plainly visible on my car's passenger seat. I held the keys to the house in my hand. Inside, my mother, brother, sister, uncle, and young cousin ate dinner unaware. If he'd wanted, he could have done a whole lot more damage.

He didn't. He would have killed me for eighteen dollars.

I LEARNED THREE THINGS early in my life. I learned to idolize work. I learned faith in absolute truth. And I learned to fear the Other—the foreign, the different, people like the man who robbed me.

All three were connected, and I had to unlearn each of them to solve for why. To explain them, however, I need to get into some history, because these three lessons are interwoven with a Lebanese diaspora of which my family is a part.

Thirty years before the robbery, under that Middle Eastern sun, more than eighteen dollars lay at stake. The history of the Lebanese Civil War is so complex that Robert Fisk's 2002 account of it, *Pity the Nation*, spans 750 pages. At one level, however, the Lebanese Civil War was a religious conflict, pitting Christians, like my family, against Muslims, like their friends.

The Levant—Lebanon, Palestine, Jordan, Cyprus, and Israel—occupies a strategic post on the eastern shores of the Mediterranean, a position that has made it the site of a dozen conflicts since the fall of the Ottoman Empire. When allied militaries defeated the Ottomans at the end of World War I and divided the empire, the Levant proved particularly problematic. Initially, the British field marshal created a short-lived Occupied Enemy Territory Administration, whose rule was allotted to British, French, and Arab administrators. At San Remo in 1920, the Enemy split in two; Britain retained Palestine, and the French took what is now Syria and Lebanon.

Because of where it sits, the Levant has always been a pastiche of cultures, languages, and religions. The Arab conquest of the seventh century cemented Islam's dominance, but large pockets of ethno-religious groups like Christians, Druze, Jews, and Kurds pepper the region.

This religious diversity is most pronounced in Lebanon.[1] In 1956, in the Lebanon of my parents' youth, 55 percent of the population was Christian, 44 percent Muslim, and the remainder a mix of adherents to Jewish, Baha'i, and other faiths.[2] Although my family comes from the Christian sector, my mother grew up in a Muslim-predominant part of Beirut, and my father's boyhood village was split evenly between Christians and Muslims.

Christian dominance in Lebanon's demography is no accident. The French created the state of Greater Lebanon specifically as a bastion for Christians in the otherwise chiefly Muslim Levant. Most Lebanese Christians are Maronites, a denomination aligned with, but separate from, the Roman Catholic Church.*

My family is not. My parents grew up within the Melkite Greek Catholic Church, a smaller, Eastern rite sect that claims lineage from Antioch, the city where the word *Christian* was first used to describe followers of an itinerant Jewish carpenter

---

* Lebanon's Maronites follow the teachings of a fourth-century Syriac hermit monk. The head of the Maronite Church, called the Patriarch of Antioch and the Whole Levant, is elected from within the Maronite religious without overt influence from the Roman Catholic Church. Upon his election, however, he requests—and is granted—recognition by the pope, who responds by making him a cardinal.

prophet. Melkites and Maronites tended to view each other with mutual distrust and disdain.

Six years after the colonial powers conferred at San Remo, the Republic of Lebanon was declared, cementing the hegemony of its Christian majority. The three key government positions were constitutionally split along religious lines: the president was to be a Maronite Christian, the prime minister a Sunni Muslim (selected by the Christian president), and the speaker of the Parliament a Shia Muslim.

This arrangement lasted exactly one administration. In 1932, two Maronite politicians campaigned for the presidency, along with Sheikh Muhammad al-Jisr, Tripoli's Muslim leader. Fearing he would lose to his rival, one of the Maronite politicians withdrew in favor of Jisr, precipitating a constitutional crisis. Lebanon's French overlords responded by suspending the constitution, thereby keeping Christians in artificial power.[3]

Lebanon declared independence from France on November 22, 1943. When the last French soldier departed in 1946, he left a Christian majority in firm control of the country's political system.

ALTHOUGH LEBANON'S NEXT HALF decade was mostly peaceful, this wasn't true in the rest of the Levant. After Britain's mandate over Palestine ended in 1947, the United Nations Partition Plan for Palestine split that country into two states: a consolidated Jewish state, and a noncontiguous Arab state whose borders approximated the current West Bank, Gaza, parts of southern Israel, Jaffa, and the region around Acre that borders Lebanon.[4]

Surprising exactly nobody, the partition plan proved unpopular. An intercommunal war between Arab and Jewish militias—which began a day after the UN passed the plan— became, after the declaration of Israeli independence in 1948, a cross-national war between Israel and the Arab states.[5]

Streams of refugees overwhelmed the northern border, settling in Lebanon and shifting its demographic and sectarian balance—a shift that threatened Maronite hegemony.

They wouldn't let go easily, however. In 1952, Camille Chamoun, another Maronite Christian, became the country's president. Toward the end of his six-year term, he intimated that he would amend the constitution, which did not allow sequential presidential terms, to try to stand for a second one.[6]

Amid growing violence, including a coup attempt by an Egyptian-backed group of left-wing Sunni pan-Arabists, Chamoun cunningly turned to the United States for help. Its new Eisenhower Doctrine had committed America to providing military and economic aid for any Middle Eastern country threatened by "overt armed aggression from any nation controlled by International Communism."[7] That became Chamoun's play: his upstanding, Christian, democratic regime was being attacked by Muslim communists.

Fourteen thousand American troops landed in Lebanon for Operation Blue Bat. Skirmishes turned to clashes, riots turned bloody. And Pierre Gemayel appeared.

IF THERE'S ONE MAN whose philosophy of the Other infiltrated into my family, it was Pierre Gemayel. He and his Phalange militia played an outsize role in the ensuing civil war and in my family's complex wartime hagiography. My parents hated him—and he, they say, hated the Melkites—but his nationalist ideas insinuated themselves into my family's consciousness.

When Bashir, Pierre's son and president-elect, was assassinated in 1982, the Christian Lebanese diaspora in Dallas sat vigil. A portrait of the slain man lay against the altar at a downtown church. My family paid its hushed respects. They had hoped Bashir's aborted presidency would usher in peace.

What I didn't know at that vigil—I was too young and too bored, the church too warm and too quiet—was that the man on the altar was no saint.

I didn't know how insidiously his family had co-opted religion for political gain. I didn't know that his father had modeled the Phalange after Italian Fascism. I didn't know that the militia wore brown shirts and adopted Hitler's straight-armed salute.[8] And I didn't know that they would avenge Bashir's assassination by massacring 3,500 Palestinian Muslims at the Sabra and Shatila refugee camps two days later, all under Israel's guidance.

Here's what I did know. I knew that Gemayel had told us that Christian Lebanese were different. I knew that he—and my family—espoused Phoenicianism, a philosophy that taught that we weren't Arab. Instead, Christian Lebanese descended from the Phoenicians.[9] The same seafaring traders who developed the world's first alphabet were our forebears—and not the forebears of Arab Muslims.

These are troubling assertions built on fraught history. They're also how Pierre Gemayel consolidated power. He adopted them as a key plank in the Phalangist platform, using them to bolster a staunch nationalism. By setting his people apart, he could paint his enemies—pan-Arabists, leftists, and Muslims—as less than. Dirty. Other.

It worked. Gemayel and the Phalangists chiseled out a position of ethnic superiority, and we, while hating everything the

Phalangists did, grew up knowing we were set apart. We had more in common with Europeans than with our darker Arab neighbors.

THERE'S SOME TRUTH TO Gemayel's assertion of European and Phoenician identity. A small genetic study of ninety-nine Lebanese people showed that a large portion of our DNA traces directly back to Canaanite Phoenician traders.[10] But intermarriage after the Arab conquest means we aren't pure-blooded.

My mother's family can also trace its lineage to an Irish merchant who came to the Middle East to ply his trade while Crusaders crusaded. And in Lebanon's more affluent sectors, French education and culture supplanted Arab culture after World War I.

Her family comes from those affluent sectors. She was born in Beirut, the second-youngest child of a prosperous, landowning, Christian family. She and her six siblings grew up in French schools, living a life buttressed by domestic help and the trappings of wealth.

My father came from the other side of Christian Lebanon. The second-youngest son of an eight-person family in the northern Lebanese village of Fakeha, my dad grew up in the shadow of Roman ruins. He was educated at Arabic-speaking boarding schools. When he and my mother met, he had to learn French to woo her; she had to learn Arabic to understand him.

Their story was a personification of the divisions splitting this patchwork country, divisions that would come to a head a few months after I was born in 1974. In coastal Sidon, Camille Chamoun—the guy who convinced Eisenhower to send American troops into Lebanon, and one of Gemayel's staunchest allies—decided to monopolize the fishing industry. His takeover was opposed by Maarouf Saad, a left-leaning, exceptionally popular Muslim politician with ties to Egypt and Palestine.

Chamoun offered Saad's unionized fishermen higher pay if they'd break ranks and cross to his side. They refused. Saad responded with a general strike. He was repaid with a sniper's bullet. He died within a week.[11]

Six weeks later, Pierre Gemayel attended a baptism in a Greek Orthodox church in East Beirut. Phalangists erected protective roadblocks outside the church. When a bus carrying Palestinian Muslims refused to divert around the roadblocks, the militia killed the driver. An hour later, as the baptism ended, two cars plastered with pro-Palestinian posters opened fire, killing the father of the baptized child and three of Gemayel's bodyguards. Gemayel survived unscathed.

That was all it took. The powder keg burst. The fifteen-year civil war it ignited would kill 6 percent of the country's population and would only end when Syria occupied Lebanon. Neighbors became enemies. The ethos of the Other that Gemayel had cultivated turned lethal, and many of the most brutal killings were committed by Christians.

ONCE THE WAR STARTED, a fair number of Lebanon's Christians—especially those who were better-off and European educated—fled. My family is part of this diaspora.

After boarding school, my dad graduated with an engineering degree from the American University of Beirut and moved to the suburbs of Chicago for his PhD. For the rest of his life, he spoke bleakly about those grim Illinois winters, in no small part because he put himself through grad school working as a stevedore on Chicago's docks.

He then moved to Dallas for a job with Texas Instruments. According to family lore, projects he worked on turned into antilock brakes and TI's first calculator. He'd never tell you that, though. The man never spoke about his accomplishments.

He held three patents: one for an improved typewriter daisy wheel,[12] one for a method for the confidential transfer of facsimiles,[13] and one for a clock[14] to indicate "the direction of a favoured place, such as Mecca, and . . . the hour of the various Islamic prayers."

My dad was as inquisitive and entrepreneurial as he was taciturn. He worked hard and found solace in his garage woodshop. And he quickly tired of the Dallas dating scene. He decided his wife, whoever she was, still lived in Lebanon. So, he flew home.

He was thirty-one when he met my mother. She fell in love with his laugh.

They got married in 1972 and bought a house in a predominantly Muslim part of Beirut. By 1975, when a just-baptized infant lost his father to a firefight at a Greek Orthodox church, I was barely a year old.

Over the next year, checkpoints metastasized across the road between Beirut and Fakeha, a rash of semiofficial barricades, manned by a splintering constellation of warring militias. It was here that, under the Middle Eastern sun, and backed by nationalist fervor and an ethos of the Other, a soldier pointed his gun at my mother's head.

We were on our way north, from Beirut to Fakeha. The first half of that two-hour drive went through Christian-controlled parts of the country. Our car passed unhindered.

Once we entered the Muslim-controlled north, however, we hit the checkpoints. At each, my father would leave the car, show his ID, open the trunk to inspection, and introduce the militia to his pregnant wife and one-year-old child. Lebanese ID cards listed the holder's religion and denomination; they served as shibboleth, allowing safe passage through friendly checkpoints and harassment at the others.

After five consecutive stops, he got frustrated.

"Look, I *just* showed everyone my car," he told the soldier.

"Get out," the man replied.

"But—"

"Out."

There wasn't a lot he could say. The soldiers knew this.

They also knew he had a pregnant wife and young son in the back seat. A second soldier trained his weapon at us.

"Get out or I shoot her."

My dad got out. They confiscated his ID and herded him toward a dozen other men whose cars, wives, and families awaited them beside the road.

My dad never spoke about this episode, but to hear my mother tell it, his escape wasn't guaranteed. Hours passed; more men joined the crowd. As the sun set, one of the militia asked my dad where he was headed.

"To Fakeha to see my mother," he replied.

"Listen. Take it from me. Turn around and go back home."

As he said this, the Lebanese Army opened fire on the checkpoint. In the chaotic churn, he ran.

Back to the car, back to his wife and child. And back the way he came. South, to the parts of the country where people looked, talked, and thought like us.

That night, the militia decapitated anyone left at the checkpoint.

*   *   *

MY PARENTS NEVER BELIEVED they'd leave Lebanon for good. My dad may have barely escaped execution, but, to them, this was all just another violent outburst between Christian and Muslim, between white and brown. They'd seen it before. It would be terrifying but short-lived.

But after the checkpoint incident, my father was now an ID-less Christian living in Muslim Beirut. They had no choice. When they packed their children—now two of us—into a plane flying west, they figured they'd be back in a year. Two, at most.

Along with their children, they also packed three ideological stowaways with them, the three ideas I'd have to unlearn. The most insidious is Gemayel's ethos of the Other.

In Texas, my parents orchestrated an uneasy balance for their immigrant kids: weekends of homeschooled Arabic and French lessons in tenuous coexistence with a strong push to assimilate. They would chastise us when our English didn't sound like that of Dan Rather, Peter Jennings, or Alex Trebek.

And we assimilated. Starting in the sixth grade, my brother and I attended an all-boys Catholic school run by Hungarian monks. My graduating class of twenty-eight had one South Asian student, one East Asian student.

And me. We were the diversity, but if you asked me in high school, I couldn't have told you that. Until 1990, I was white.* I had internalized Gemayel's divisive philosophy. It fit with my new Texan home. And my family reinforced it—sometimes explicitly.

---

* To be fair, in the eyes of the United States government, I still am. Although airport security takes a lurid interest in my bags every time I fly, the US Census specifically instructs people of Middle Eastern descent to check "white" on their census forms.

I had my first serious relationship in college. Adele is from Singapore; you'll see her again in a few chapters, but I bring her up here because of what happened the day my parents first met her. Poor Adele—she had no idea what she was walking into when she ran into my family during their campus visit. Always the consummate hostess, my mother invited her to a very pleasant lunch that day. We got pancakes.

Things turned less cordial that night, after Adele left. In their hotel room, my parents handed down an unambiguous lesson in the ethos of the Other.

If we were to date, they told their three children, we had to adhere to a hierarchy of peoples. If we couldn't find ourselves a good Christian Lebanese partner, white Christians were okay. East Asians like Adele were third best.

God forbade anyone else.

We protested. They told us not to be naive. They used to have friends across religious and ethnic lines, once. Then the war happened, and friends killed each other. The only people we could trust were our kind.

We're all formed by—and have to unlearn—histories we don't choose. My parents, who have since vehemently disavowed this hierarchy, were formed by theirs just as their history became part of mine.

LIKE EVERYONE ELSE IN Texas in August 1990, I watched, rapt, as America insinuated ourselves into the first Gulf War, injecting our armies into a conflict that didn't involve us.

I watched as news anchors breathlessly narrated the full might of our air forces imposing our politics on a country that suffered— we were told—under a brutal regime. The short-haired Texan oil baron turned president assured us it would be quick and safe. We would liberate the Others (and their oil). We wouldn't lose any of Us.

I also watched, rapt, as a classmate insinuated his red convertible into a prime spot in the school's parking lot the next morning. His car's stereo tore the August air with The Cure's "Killing an Arab."

Staring down the barrel at the Arab on the ground.
I can see his open mouth, but I hear no sound.

On August 3, 1990, I became Other.

My family's Phoenicianism evaporated, and with it their insistences that we keep ourselves apart, their assertions that we were separate, purer, whiter, more European, and more Christian. The Arabs I'd learned to shun, the ones I'd learned to Other, were now me.

No matter how addicted I am to donuts, no matter how many times my parents corrected me when I didn't speak Dan Rather's English, I still got raw lamb with bulgur as a birthday cake.

It didn't matter that my Arabic is terrible. It didn't matter that my French is, at best, stuck in stilted language-lab phrases about finding the nearest toilet. My family has its own recipe for hummus as thick as my dad's accent. The tenuous American veneer we'd built shattered that morning.

I had spent nearly my entire life in Texas. I stood for the Pledge of Allegiance. I could play Jimi Hendrix's guitar-solo version of the national anthem. I went to church every Wednesday and twice on Sunday. I believed in the might and the right of America.

And I am an Arab. That August, my home attacked my people. Soldiers who talked like me attacked people who looked like me, and other people wrote songs about it. People who looked like my friends dropped bombs on people who spoke like my uncles. They annihilated people who dressed like my grandmother, people who lived in flat-topped houses and hung their laundry out to dry and slept on roofs under the stars on nights when the air was too hot and too still.

That August night, I became Other.

Chapter 2

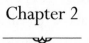

Truth may be vital, but without love it is unbearable.

—JONATHAN PRYCE AS POPE FRANCIS,

THE TWO POPES

FINLAY GRAHAM CUTS AN imposing figure in Lebanon's Christian history. He was also my best friend's grandfather.

Scottish by descent, always impeccably dressed, Grandpa Finlay decided to become a missionary to Lebanon while midflight over the Middle East as a World War II Royal Air Force pilot. He spent four decades in my parents' country, its first Southern Baptist missionary.

Between the end of the war and 1986, when he and his wife Julia finally retired to Texas, he founded a Baptist seminary, the Beirut Baptist School, and the first Lebanese Baptist church. "Today," wrote the author of his obituary, "there are more Baptist churches in Lebanon than there were individual believers when the Grahams got started." According to his colleague, Nancie Wingo, "They all have their roots back in that first church."[1]

Grandpa Finlay tempered his strong will with a penchant

for corny Scottish sayings. His was a forbidding presence, meekness surrounding an iron core.

He'd already retired to Texas by the time he handed his grandson's pimpled, introverted friend a list of ten rules for living. I wish I still had Finlay's ten rules. Until I left for college, the torn piece of paper he'd typed them on lived pinned above my desk, a ragged distillation of a Scottish Christian missionary's work ethic. I learned those ten rules by heart back then, but I can only remember the fifth:

Wear out in the Lord's service. Don't rust out.

The inherent goodness of work, crystallized in ten syllables. It was Grandpa Finlay's rule, and it's the second ideological stowaway my parents brought over from Lebanon.

On its face, it doesn't seem all that bad. Work. Self-reliance. Grit. Determination. This stowaway holds well-deserved power. My family espoused its gospel. It took my dad from Chicago's docks to Texas Instruments' labs to his own company. It allowed my mother and father to rebuild a family in a country whose language neither spoke well.

It's a gospel I also internalized. Wear out, don't rust out. Work, like your father worked. Be a productive member of society. Raise a successful family. Start a successful company. Chart a successful career. Be a successful missionary.

Work, because work purifies. It redeems. Succeed, don't rust.

My parents sent me to that all-boys school run by Hungarian monks specifically because I wasn't working at our

neighborhood grade school. I spent weekdays with my mis-
behaving butt stuffed into a trash can in the corner of Sister
Viola's first-grade classroom, or wilting under Miss Houston's
tobaccoed ennui. And my parents weren't about to raise a
delinquent.

At a school where black-and-white-clad monks glided
through muted, ceramic-tiled halls, I learned to work. Father
Mathew's vestigial belief in corporal punishment, Father Gregory's penchant for the dramatic, and Father Roch's procliv-
ity for dissecting minute aspects of New Testament theology
taught me to work, and work saved me.

I can be ruinously shy. I'm terrified of risk, as you'll soon
discover. I wore sweatshirts even in the hottest Texas summers,
because the switch from sweatshirts to short sleeves was too
scary. Besides, sweatshirts were safe. They hid my short, puny
frame. I'd rather wither in a sweatshirt than under the harsh
judgment of my grade school peers.

At the all-boys Catholic school, I grew out of those sweatshirts and grew into work. Through work, I discovered I could
be someone. It wouldn't make me popular, but at least it could
protect me from my shyness. It wouldn't admit me to the inner
circles, but work could save me from bullying. No one's going
to bully someone whose notes they rely on.

I threw myself into it. I became good at work. The harder
I worked, the more I gained an identity: I learned that I was
nothing if I wasn't the best at something. To be good is not
good enough if you dream of being great, they say. I dreamed
of being the best, because being the best was what my family
demanded.

I was born again in Grandpa Finlay's fifth rule. My dad didn't escape death at a Lebanese checkpoint for his son to be mediocre. Only mediocre people rusted out. And I refused to rust.

BOTH IDEOLOGICAL STOWAWAYS MY family brought with them—the ethos of the Other and the ethos of Work—anneal under a third: faith. Just as I had to disassemble the first two before I could find my why, I wouldn't discover true worship until I dismantled the faith of my childhood.

My parents raised their children as Roman Catholics. It was the closest they could find to their Melkite Christian Lebanese upbringing. In the eighth grade, Arnaldo, Grandpa Finlay's grandson, invited me to a summer camp run by the conservative Evangelical church he and his family attended.

That camp scared the hell out of me. Literally.

On the final night, after a week of haranguing his pubescent audience with Saint Paul's writings, the preacher detailed God's "white-hot anger" toward us, his "hatred" toward anyone who did not accept Jesus as their Lord and Savior. His face reddened as he spat those four words. Hatred. White. Hot. Anger.

Father Roch, Father Mathew, and Father Gregory had taught me an omnipotent God. Now, this dark-haired preacher pulled verses I'd never heard from the word of that same God. He taught me about hell. He taught me that the omnipotent God obeyed the ethos of the Other, that the eyes of the Almighty saw only two types of people: those who accepted him and those who didn't. And he taught me that the latter were predestined to an eternity of white-hot anger.

I cried. I prayed terrified prayers. That night, I was born again.

I moved from the strictures and traditions of Catholicism to the strictures and traditions of something that styled itself unstrictured and anti-tradition.

I started attending Arnaldo's small church. I listened as another dark-haired preacher told us that only his style of Christianity was right, and that anyone else—especially those idolatrous Catholics—didn't truly worship God.

And I learned to separate the world. I learned dichotomy—the saved and the unsaved, the chosen and the rest, Us and Other. I learned God's wrath toward the Other. The chosen—and we alone—knew right from wrong.

I learned to traffic in, and to worship, absolute truths. Pity the soul who disagreed.

I AM THE SON of a refugee family. I learned life from a resolute Scottish missionary. I was schooled at the feet of Hungarian monks. I worshipped at a church that claimed ultimate truth. My people are people of grit. We keep our heads down, our eyes forward. We don't dream, don't question. We do what we're told. We brook no discussion. We work. And we don't quit.

I grew up believing in universal truths. The ethics of my youth were self-perpetuating. They felt no need to defend themselves. Their thetic, theocratic claims imbued in them an air of unquestioned permanence. Their truths, I was told, would set me free.

They were exactly what I had to unlearn to solve for why. Because if a truth doesn't set you free, is the problem with you or with that truth?

Chapter 3

The man who will not act till he knows all will never act at all.

—JIM ELLIOT

I NEVER WANTED TO be a doctor.

Drunk crickets trace neater paths through sand than I do with pen on paper. In grade school, I was a mediocre student—except in penmanship. I almost failed that. Sister Viola—she of the butts-in-wastebasket punishments—and her successors sent my parents desperate entreaties to fix their son's handwriting. Thankfully, cursive skill doesn't play the role in my life they said it would.

To my parents, however, my penmanship was proof: their son was destined for medicine.

"No!" I'd respond. "I don't want to be a doctor. I want to be a rock star!" Because what little boy doesn't want to be a rock star?

More than anything, I wanted to play music. I grew my hair out to match the guitarists I admired. I took to wearing all black, adorning my neck with massive crosses fashioned out of rusty nails.

I fantasized about being on a stage in front of thousands, under the blue lights and the smoke machines, drums behind me, monitor amps in front of me. When I wasn't thinking about anything else, I imagined a single spotlight reflecting off my guitar, the keen of its strings as my band played the songs I was destined to write.

But let's be honest. I was never going to be a rock star. The first time my parents heard the album my high school band recorded, eddies of unrealized hope circled their faces. My father fought to keep his eyes steady, unwidened. He didn't blink.

"What...is this?" he asked, and, in those three words, he leveraged the full force of history, of filial devotion, of a family that had toiled the fields of Fakeha so that they could, what? Have their offspring dither his life away recording heavy metal music?

My mother said nothing.

To be fair, the album was terrible.

It didn't stop me. I played my guitar constantly. Obsessed with Petra, a Christian rock band all of whose CDs I still own, I learned every note their guitarist wrote. The way Bob Hartman bent his strings, I bent mine. His timing, his syncopation, his melodic choices—they became mine too. Those dreams of being onstage, a single spotlight shining on my guitar, were dreams of playing with Bob.

When I learned to drive, I would tap out the rhythm of his songs on my steering wheel, lost in the fantasy that the band would pull their white van alongside my car (because they obviously cruised the streets of Dallas in a white van). The drummer would notice the awkward teenager drubbing the steering wheel of the car to his left. Through the window and across two lanes, he'd recognize it—wait! He's drumming our songs! Before long, I'd be onstage with Bob.

Not content to rely on chance encounters with white vans, I covered my bases. Every couple of years, I sent Petra letters. I reminded them of my guitar-playing skills and offered my services, should the band ever need them. I sent the dot-matrix printouts folded into carefully addressed envelopes to Nashville. Petra still hasn't responded.

OTHER DAYS, I WANTED to be a philosopher. Because what little boy doesn't want to be a philosopher? If I wasn't going to be a rock star, getting paid just to think—and to tell other people how to think—sounded perfect.

Truth is, though, I wanted to be a linguist, because what I really wanted to be was a missionary.

I grew up reading the stories of missionaries: people like Bruce Olson, an American missionary from Minnesota; like Hudson Taylor, a British missionary to China; or like Jim Elliot, the modern-day martyr whose life captivated young Christians in my generation.

Their journeys fit every ethos I grew up under. They were men of faith. They worked hard. They preached to the Other, convincing them to abandon their beliefs in favor of absolute truth. They didn't rust. These men led impressive lives, lives I wanted.

Bruce worked in Latin America. In the early 1960s, the Barí people in Colombia and Venezuela clashed with oil companies who planned to drill on their land. The Barí number in the few thousands. They speak a vulnerable, indigenous language and live in an economy based primarily on the cultivation and export of cacao.

Their fight captured Olson's imagination. It took him a few years—and being shot at by a few arrows—before he would live among them, a golden-haired missionary of Scandinavian descent, ensconced in a tribe that, prior to his arrival, had had vanishingly little contact with outsiders.

How he gained that access is a story in itself. The Barí are monotheistic. Their oral tradition told of a prophet who had vowed to bring them to the promised land over the mountains. They followed him, in vain: the prophet's mantle was false, and his exodus led them away from God. God, in punishment, had abandoned them.

Rejected, they didn't give up. They continued to worship the God who'd turned his back on them, hoping to shoehorn themselves into his favor. Healers chanted, people prayed, but nobody believed it would work. God had left the Barí.

The prophesies also told of hope, however, of a tall man with yellow hair who would lead them back to God. He'd do it with a banana stalk. In fact, God himself would be in that very banana stalk.

Bruce, a tall man with yellow hair, had survived their arrows. Sure, God hadn't appeared out of the banana stalk yet, but at least part of the prophecy had come true. They cautiously let him stay.

Not long after his arrival, the Barí faced a recalcitrant conjunctivitis outbreak. Despite her ministrations, the local healer couldn't overcome the epidemic of pinkeye. Olson had an idea:

he purposely infected himself, touching his fingers to the eyes of a patient and then to his own. Once infected, he visited the traditional healer and asked her to chant over him.

She did. It didn't work. He then gave her a salve he'd brought. Would she mind chanting over him again, this time after he applied the ointment to his eyes? She agreed, but only if she could also change her chant. It was possible the yellow-haired man was governed by different forces than the Barí, forces she hadn't initially accounted for.

Bruce applied the antibiotic. The healer chanted her new chant. And the infection cleared.

In a spectacular example of scientific equipoise, the traditional healer got curious. What had worked? Was it the second chant, his ointment, or both?

She tried the new chant on other Barí. It failed. She tried her chant and Olson's salve, and the outbreak ended. The yellow-haired man was onto something.

Olson parlayed his success into health centers throughout Barí villages. His strategy treated the Barí culture with a respect we in global health still haven't figured out: he brought the traditional healers into the health system as partners, instead of shuttering them. He knew his ointments were scientifically more effective than their chants, but he never let that get in the way of remembering that he was a guest.

His partner in the health centers was a man named Bobarishora. On one of their regular village walks, Bobarishora split a banana stalk lengthwise. Its tightly wound sheaves unfurled. Like a book. Like the book Olson carried that told of his God. Olson remembered the prophecy under whose protection he'd been living.

"This!" he said, pointing to his Bible. "This is God's banana stalk!"

Today, 70 percent of the Barí are Christians. I wanted to be a missionary like Bruce Olson.

OR LIKE HUDSON TAYLOR. I devoured every book I could find on Taylor. Born in 1832 to a British chemist and a Methodist lay preacher, Taylor spent fifty-one years working as a medical missionary to China. Like Olson, he went all in. On his first posting in coastal China, his dour, black English dress made people call him a "black devil."

To counter that, he adopted Chinese clothing and the common tonsure-plus-ponytail hairstyle. He also decided that coastal China presented too little of a challenge. He needed to go inland, to spread his message to people he hadn't yet reached.

Taylor lost his family to China. His daughter, Grace, died of meningitis; his two sons, Samuel and Noel, and his wife, Maria, all succumbed to cholera in the country. He never wavered.

His dedication, his ingenuity—he trained neighborhood cats to be a pest-control army—and his tenacity until his death in 1905 in Changsha all modeled the life I wanted. Grandpa Finlay would have loved Hudson Taylor.

AND THEN THERE WAS Jim Elliot. Any boy growing up in the American Protestant church in the 1980s and 1990s knew about Jim and Elisabeth Elliot. More than Olson, more than Taylor, we dreamed of being like Jim. We prayed nightly for a relationship like his and Elisabeth's. We read their books. We quoted their writing. If Elisabeth came to speak, we moved heaven and earth to sit at her feet.

Unshakable pillars of the turn-of-the-century Protestant zeitgeist, Jim and Elisabeth wielded a gentle power over us. "He is no fool," Jim had written in his journals, "who gives what he cannot keep to gain that which he cannot lose."[1] We memorized this. We set it to music.

Had social media been a thing, we would have plastered it on our feeds, white text over tastefully blurred pictures of mountain sunsets.

Jim and Elisabeth's marriage lasted only three years, because Jim died chasing his purpose. Drawn—called, he'd say—to the Huaorani, Jim and a small group of like-minded missionaries arrived in Ecuador in 1952. The Huaorani were known for a vicious ruthlessness toward outsiders. Their neighbors called them Auca, a Quechua word meaning *savage*.

After initial contact with the tribe by air, Jim and his four companions decided to build a base downriver. Initial friendly encounters bolstered their confidence. By 1956, they were ready to visit the Huaorani in person.

The Huaorani weren't. On January 8, 1956, a dozen Huaorani warriors attacked the camp, killing all five missionaries.

I'M NOT GOING TO lie. Writing about nineteenth- and twentieth-century missionaries in the twenty-first century is difficult. Today, we're acutely aware of the detrimental effect missionaries can have—and have had—on the cultures to which they felt called.

We know how destructive mission trips can be. We know the unwitting arrogance and hubris that can define the missionary impulse. As I write this chapter, followers of a Tongan Christian missionary to the Australian outback are actively setting fire to Aboriginal artifacts they view as satanic.[2]

We also know how deeply rooted missionary work can be in the same ethos of the Other that I grew up with. My goal here isn't to defend or to debate the work of these three men, and hundreds like them. I tell their stories because they are my stories. I aspired to be these men. How they lived their lives is how I intended to live Grandpa Finlay's fifth rule. Taylor and Elliot sacrificed their lives for their convictions. Nothing could be more noble.

Crucially, none of them worked in Africa, which was serendipitous, because I never wanted to work on that continent. I'd grown up to view it as a single, monolithic, dirty place, hot, dry, and infested with bugs.

I was determined to be a missionary, but on my own terms. During a college mission trip to a Palestinian refugee camp in Jordan, I committed myself to modeling Hudson Taylor's life specifically. On the flat-topped roof of our homestay, a friend and I leaned over the balustrade, watching the sun set over a dusty city. I told him I wanted to do this for the rest of my life. I was going to be a missionary in Asia. Like Hudson Taylor.

That night, he and I prayed that God would never send me to Africa.

DAYDREAMS NOTWITHSTANDING, PETRA WASN'T ever going to drive by in a white van and hire me on the streets of Dallas. But Jim and Bruce and Hudson? Theirs was an attainable life, an inspiring life. If, at the end of my own life, my grave looked like theirs, I would have achieved my purpose.

Linguistics would be my ticket. It would take me into Asian jungles. I would disappear into Papua New Guinea for decades. I'd create the writing system for a language that had never been written. I would translate the Bible; I'd codify the oral history of a people threatened with extinction; I'd teach them the right way to live; and I'd return only after my work was done. Or I'd die trying. This was my dream.

Linguistics still fascinates me—the sounds we make, how tone confers meaning, why some languages use alphabets and others use syllabaries, how words evolve across time, and why Yoda sounds weird to just about everyone.* I still sometimes read linguistics textbooks before going to bed.

But, I'm the firstborn son of an immigrant family. And firstborn sons of immigrant families really only have three options: doctor, lawyer, or failure.

In her controversial book *Battle Hymn of the Tiger Mother*, Amy Chua took unapologetic possession of a caricature: Asian parents brooked no foolishness from their children. She defended the demands she and her husband put on their children, claiming these demands in childhood led to success in adulthood.

---

* Whether it was intentional on George Lucas's part or not, Yoda's syntax belongs to a distinctive, and incredibly rare, linguistic typology. Most English sentences adopt a subject-verb-object (or SVO) structure: "I drew a tree," for example. *I* is the subject, *drew* the verb, and *tree* the object. This is the second-most-common structure globally; 42 percent of the world's languages have an SVO typology. A bit more common are SOV languages, like Korean or Japanese.

Yoda doesn't adhere to either of these structures. When he says, "Much to learn, you still have," he's using an OSV—object-subject-verb—typology. In the wild, fewer than 1 percent of the world's languages are OSV, and all come from the Amazon basin.

Interestingly, we English speakers do occasionally use an OSV structure when we want to emphasize certain parts of a sentence. Consider the lyrics to the song "Friendly Persuasion": "Thee I love, more than the meadows so green and still." Here, "Thee I love" is OSV, just as Yoda would have wanted it.

East Asian parents don't have a corner on the tiger mother market. We Lebanese hold our own. Being a rock star, a linguist, a philosopher, or a missionary? Not even worth consideration. My choices were clear: I would carry on my father's business, or I would go into medicine, the law, or some other respectable entrepreneurial endeavor of my own.

Full stop.

I didn't want to be a lawyer or a businessman, but I liked science. My high school biology teacher knew how to breathe delight into his subject. He encouraged exploration; he welcomed questions; he taught me to think.

So, if it wasn't going to be linguistics or philosophy or music, then it would have to be science. Still, I didn't go quietly. On our tour of universities, my dad insisted on visiting every biology lab he could find. With the visceral disinterest of a seventeen-year-old, I stared blankly at the protein gels or the genetically modified fruit fly colonies that were supposed to cure cancer.

I didn't care. I was going to be a linguist-philosopher-rock-star-missionary. Fruit flies? Gels? Curing cancer? Completely banal.

My poor dad. I forced him to reject so many majors during college, to torpedo so many potential career paths before I finally succumbed. I can't imagine the conversations he and my mother must have had after every phone call. "I found it, Dad! I'm going to major in music composition! No? How's psychology—that works, right?"

Each time, he returned to one maxim: no child of his would study a subject whose "only purpose is to perpetuate itself." His words. Music, philosophy, and linguistics fell under that aegis.

Reluctantly, I capitulated.

* · * · *

FULLY 95 PERCENT OF the students graduating from molecular biology where I went to school in the mid-1990s went on to medical training. I may never have wanted to be a doctor, but, every other dream denied, I had no reason *not* to follow them.

What a strange disrespect for my values that stance is: not wanting to be a doctor wasn't a strong enough reason not to be a doctor. As a college senior, though, I didn't know better. I had internalized the ethos of Work, so doctoring made sense. It was respectable. It satisfied my elders. It had value.

I took the required courses, eked out a passable score on the MCAT, and applied to twenty-five different medical schools.

Of which twenty-three rejected me. They saw what I couldn't. Despite my superficial assurances that being a doctor would fulfill all my childhood dreams, my heart wasn't in it, and they sensed it.

They looked behind the tightly crafted personal statements to the ennui that undergirded them. I couldn't yet articulate that I only applied to medical school because it was acceptable, because it was safe, and because it fit my family's ethos, but they heard it anyway.

"Success for you," their rejections said, "can't be found in our halls. Look elsewhere."

I didn't listen.

LET ME TAKE A small detour here to talk about success.

Success looks different for everyone. True success is individual, and it's only found at the end of a life lived in service of why.

As a culture, however, we espouse a narrow, monolithic

definition of success, one that fits Grandpa Finlay's fifth rule. According to the story we're fed, success looks like financial security, a respectable job, and a happy family. It's such a trenchant story because it simplifies major life decisions. It keeps us from having to solve for why.

And if we don't have to do the hard work of solving, we're free to let life happen to us. We can measure success through tangible outcomes: promotions, money, children, houses. Because this definition's simplicity is so alluring, its tendrils insinuate themselves everywhere.

The problem with this monolithic definition lies not in the things it makes us pursue—there's nothing wrong with money, career success, or a fulfilling family life—but in the fact that, unless these things are *actually* our why, they end up feeling like a trap.

This kind of success charts a wide, smooth, and well-populated path through the banality of privilege, to a conclusion we're not convinced we actually want. Like lidocaine to our psyches, it numbs us to why.

The wide, smooth, anodyne path is like a moving sidewalk at an airport, as safe as it is boring. It'll get you to a destination, but once you're on it it's almost impossible to get off. And unless that destination is one you actually want, the moving sidewalk does you no good.

On the moving sidewalk, we go to school, sometimes to college, sometimes to graduate school. Then we dive headlong into the churn of a three-decade career. Somewhere in there, we find a spouse to whom we may or may not stay married, have kids to whom we may or may not be devoted, and buy a house whose mortgage we may or may not pay off. And then we exit the churn, bruised, battered, beige, and—sometimes—financially secure. In the words of Dennis Merritt Jones, we "endure until we exit the planet."[3]

I felt this in medicine. Doctors trace a prescribed arc from cradle to grave. We kill ourselves to do well in high school so we can win admission to a competitive university, where we kill ourselves to do well (again) so we can apply for medical school. Once we get in, our careers become remarkably pre-fab. Medical school for four years, residency for three to five, maybe a fellowship for another few years, and then practice for thirty. Whether we work for ourselves or join a larger hospital network, we whir through three decades of active clinical life, seeing dozens of patients a day, five days a week. Then we retire with a nice house in a nice retirement community with golf buddies we sometimes like and occasional visits from our grandchildren.

Unless medicine is our why—which, let me be clear, it is for many—we add spice only to the margins. Maybe we do research on the weekends. Maybe we go into administration. Maybe we teach. At the core, however, every doctor's life looks similar, and for good reason: medicine's prefab arc leads almost inexorably to financial security, a respectable job, and the banality of privilege.

Medicine has a cotton candy draw, wispy, sweet, ephemeral. To a college senior without a clear sense of his why and without the courage to stand up for where he thought he wanted his life to go, however, it's ultimately lethal.

Had I been honest with myself, I wouldn't have applied to medical school. Had I done the work of solving for why, I wouldn't have started on the moving sidewalk. And had I been honest in my med school applications, I wouldn't have gotten in anywhere. I wouldn't have fooled two schools into accepting me.

Instead, I said the things I was supposed to say, wrote the personal statement I was supposed to write, and tried to convince the admissions committee that, yes, I really did dream of being a doctor. I made majestic, far-reaching statements about both my potential future and my inner landscape, all with fingers crossed—hoping they would reject me so at least I could say I'd tried.

I could articulate none of this in the spring of 1996, as I taped twenty-three medical school rejection letters to the walls of my dorm room. All I knew was that medical school satisfied the obligations of firstborn sons of immigrant families, and, maybe, if I got lucky, I could still play music on the side.

Chapter 4

*In one of those stars, I shall be living. In one of them,
I shall be laughing. And so it will be as if all the stars
were laughing when you look at the sky at night.*

—ANTOINE DE SAINT-EXUPÉRY

IT WOULDN'T BE FAIR to write about my slide onto the moving sidewalk without talking about the single most life-altering event in my story.

Over 90 percent of us outlive our parents.[1] Pretty much all of us will bury at least one parent. And none of us is ever prepared for it. In the spring of 1996, two weeks before my college graduation, I wasn't prepared either.

My father and I were very close. Despite how strict he was, that taciturn, mustached, heavily accented tinkerer just got me. Two introverts in a home of extroverts. An electrical engineer turned business owner, he had a knack for science, for math, and for challenging questions.

He lived a quiet life. I saw him cry exactly twice: once when his mother died, and once when our family faced bankruptcy. That was also the only time I saw him drink alone, at the dinner table, a glass of opaque white arak in his left hand, his head heavy on his right.

Everything started with the kidney stone that wasn't a kidney stone. Non-Hodgkin's lymphoma primarily affects people over the age of sixty. My dad was fifty-four. He lived healthy, swam laps every night until it got too cold out, never smoked, rarely drank, ate well, and took no medications. Cancer doesn't care.

For a bit, things looked good. After successful surgery and adjuvant treatment, the doctors declared him cancer-free. Lulled by a misguided optimism toward parental immortality, I—selfishly—begged my parents for the opportunity to spend the next summer doing research in college instead of home with a convalescing father. As I battled the same protein gels I'd sneered at four years prior, lymphoma battled its way back into his body.

My dad returned to the hospital in April of 1996 with a pneumonia that wasn't a pneumonia. Back then, bone marrow transplantation was a cutting-edge treatment for lymphoma. His doctors quoted a 40 percent success rate, 60 percent mortality rate. To him, those were good enough odds. Still young, with kids just at the brink of adulthood and a wife he still loved, he knew he would be in the 40 percent.

He wasn't in the 40 percent.

By the time the bone marrow transplant had turned on its host, by the time it attacked his body, the doctors had moved him to the intensive care unit. The next week played out relentlessly, the way it would in a movie. A frenetically calm phone call from my uncle—get home now. A frantic rush to Newark airport. The prohibitive costs of last-minute travel, which the

airline would only reverse on presentation of a death certificate. The rush from the airport to the ICU to find my father
already intubated, sedated, on a ventilator. Silent.

I never got to say goodbye. As he lay there, each member
of the family got twenty minutes with him alone, to make our
peace. On May 19, 1996, I lost my rock.

GRIEF IS A BLACK, scaly monster. Disentangling its tentacles
from the next decade of my life is impossible, so I'm not going
to try.

Two weeks after my father died, I graduated from college.

The only two medical schools that accepted me were in
Texas, a state I'd hoped I'd left behind. Two weeks after my
father died, I moved back into my childhood home, an inward-
looking young man living with an outward-processing, griev-
ing family.

The sham that was my medical school essay shattered that
summer. Turns out, I really *didn't* want to be a doctor.

I wanted to be anywhere but the maroon-tiled halls of the
University of Texas Southwestern Medical School. Anywhere
but the treacly heat of a Dallas summer. Anywhere but among
cadavers in a green, fluorescent-lit anatomy lab. Anywhere but
looking at their formalin-weathered faces and their bloodlessly,
bluntly, inaptly dissected abdomens.

When the dean of students, Jim Wagner, compared the first
year of medical school to learning a new language and exploring a foreign country, when he pumped us up with breathtak-
ing stories of the rest of our lives, when he praised us for our
admission into the rarefied ranks of the life-savers, I wanted to
be in any other rank but that one.

Again, work saved me. This time, it wasn't from shyness; it was from grief.

Days shot through with caffeine, nights buried under index cards that detailed sodium's journey through the kidney's collecting system—I hated them. But they provided cover. Any minute I spent cramming the difference between succinyl-CoA synthase and succinic dehydrogenase into my brain was a minute spent away from the black, scaly monster.

I wrapped myself around medical school like it was a buoy in a rip current. But succinyl-CoA synthase never asked to be a buoy. It wasn't a good one. The more I grabbed at it, the more I floundered. The harder I thrashed, the faster I learned I wanted out.

I started medical school in August. I first tried to quit in September.

Two decades later, those medical school years feel gray, flat, and blurry. I learned, I crammed, and every day I shot up inchoate prayers. I pleaded to the God of Hudson Taylor and Jim Elliot. I begged for some path to materialize, for a miraculous exit, for anything that could rescue me without me having to rescue myself.

I needed out, but I didn't want to make the decision to leave.

Like everything else on the anodyne path, those years feel numb. And that numbness made me a coward. I wanted to quit, but I didn't want to be the quitter. I wanted to leave without leaving.

Two medical schools hadn't done me the favor of rejecting me, but maybe God could do me this solid. That way, I could say I tried. I still honored the ethos of Work, and it wasn't my fault that I failed.

I wouldn't have to remain bound, but I could abdicate responsibility for escaping. After all, the man who'd required this of me was gone—taken too early by cancer—so why was I still here?

MIRACULOUSLY, I GOT THAT opportunity. And I almost made it out.

Before my father got sick, I'd been accepted to a year-long teaching post in Singapore, through a hundred-year-old exchange program called Princeton in Asia. Every year, PiA accepts about 140 students to teaching positions throughout the continent. Most teach English, but applicants assigned to Singapore get dispensation. We teach our majors—my roommates taught everything from engineering to computer science to cinematography.

Singapore also paid better than any other PiA posting. It offered the most vacation. And Adele, whom you met in the first chapter, was Singaporean. Singapore would give us a chance to be together.

The committee agreed. I was assigned to teach biochemistry to Singaporean sixteen-year-olds.

Then my father got sick, and I withdrew. When PiA reoffered me the position at the end of my first year of medical school, I would have been a fool to turn them down. Singapore would be my escape.

Except everybody told me to turn them down.

This motif will recur in my story; it's guaranteed for anyone whose why pulls them away from their moving sidewalk. My brother, an actor and writer, has faced it, as have most physicians with nontraditional careers.

At every life-altering choice I've made, I've heard:

"This will ruin your career."

"You'll never recover."

"Any job will now see you as a flight risk."

"You're going to seem uncommitted."

"No one will take a chance on you."

"It's time for you to settle down."

"Grow up."

And you know what? This counsel isn't wrong. I'd love to be John the Baptist here—minus the locusts and the honey—a lone voice of truth crying out to people on the moving sidewalk: "These folks want to keep you down! They want to preserve order. They want to kill your dreams!"

But that's not true. People say these things out of concern. The litany of counsel does consign us to bland uniformity, but the people who espouse it do so from a place of genuine, if constricted, care.

Solving for why is risky. When recruiters and residency directors see a featureless procession of students with exactly the right credentials—students who've toed the career line, going straight from college to medical school to residency, who've spent their free summers adding hydroxyl groups to cancer drugs—then an applicant on a nontraditional path presents an unmitigated risk.

To my deans and my mentors, Singapore was that risk. Taking a year off at the wrong time to do the wrong thing in the wrong place was sheer folly.

Had I waited, though, I'd still be waiting.

Chapter 5

You rest when you're dead.

—LEE KUAN YEW, SINGAPORE'S
FOUNDING PRIME MINISTER

I FELL IN LOVE with Singapore.

Drown a pile of shaved ice in coconut milk and syrupy, brown palm sugar. Add sinuous globules of bright green rice flour and a dollop of amaranthine adzuki beans. This is chendol, a popular dessert on the Malay Peninsula, and the first thing I ate in Singapore.

At the tip of that peninsula in the South China Sea, connected to Malaysia by a narrow and perpetually congested bridge flanked with signs reminding visitors that they'll be executed for drug trafficking, sits an island only thirty-one miles across. Five and a half million people call it home. Daily, they shuttle across Singapore on a smooth, silent, driverless underground train network, reclaim land from the surrounding ocean, and eat street food cooked by dynastic hawkers in open-air markets, vestiges from before independence.

Its location on the straits that bear its name makes

Singapore's ports among the busiest in the world. Fully half of the world's crude oil and one in every five shipping containers passes through them. Every year, vessels from 123 countries on every continent drop anchor in the island's waters.

Like Lebanon, Singapore is an olio. Its food melds Malaysia, China, South India, and Britain. Its culture looks both eastward and westward. Its citizens adhere to at least eleven religions. And its stringent, authoritarian government was founded by a venerated benevolent dictator. In its colorful, pulsating streets thrum art, science, finance, commerce, and an animated exchange of ideas over char kway teow and sugarcane juice.

For me, it was also deliverance. Or, at least, my first taste of it.

I WENT TO SINGAPORE as a teacher, and Singapore's educational system first opened my eyes to what it looked like when my childhood ethos of the Other was applied to a country.

Although Singapore's educational pathways can be convoluted, when Singaporean students are in the sixth grade, they take the Primary School Leaving Examination, which immediately sets one group apart from others.[1] Students are streamed after this exam into gifted and nongifted cadres, an assignment that follows them for the rest of their educational lives.

Whether students are even allowed to attend a four-year university depends on how well they do on exams they take when they're sixteen, but these "Ordinary Level" exams aren't even available to kids who didn't do well in the sixth grade. Top-tier scorers on the O-Levels proceed to two more years of secondary school at one of nineteen prestigious junior colleges, and then sit for Advanced Level exams. Which majors they can choose depends on their A-Level results.

However, students who do poorly in the sixth grade aren't afforded the opportunity to compete for a spot in university. These students get shunted, instead, to a less prestigious academic life. Second-best students are funneled into one of several polytechnic or art institutes. In the late 1990s—this has recently changed—students graduating with their polytechnic or arts diplomas ended their education there.*

Ngee Ann Polytechnic hired me as a cellular biology and organic chemistry lab instructor. The school's sprawling campus in western Singapore is preposterously well funded: my department housed a hydroponics greenhouse, an organic chemistry laboratory, and, at the time, a dozen faculty and twice as many faculty assistants. My mentor, Mr. O. B. Chang, had a penchant for swordsmanship.

I loved Singapore as much as Mr. Chang loved his swords. I loved the food, the country, and the work. I like being an educator; I live for the split-second flash that crosses a student's face when what you've been teaching suddenly lands.

At the same time, I ran headlong into students pushing against the bounds of a punitive educational system, and I had no idea what I'd gotten myself into. My students baffled their teacher, steeped as I was in an American worldview. Since they were in the sixth grade, their educational system had told them that they were second best.

Their goal wasn't independent thought, they were told.

---

* Students who score the lowest on their sixth-grade exams aren't even eligible to sit their high school exams. They go to technical schools.

They needed to find the right answer and to regurgitate it. For some, this was great—I don't want to pretend that I spent those days in sound and fury, that I or my students railed constantly against an unjust system. But there were those who knew they could do more than the dominance structures had told them. They had academic dreams, and their sixth-grade selves had failed them. For these students, the codified reminder that they were Other, that they were somehow less than, exasperated.

I saw it. But I did nothing to fix it.

DREAMS OF BEING JIM Elliot or Hudson Taylor stood firmly on an assumption that a Lebanese kid raised in a conservative Christian, Texan household could make a home in a different country. Until Singapore, that assumption remained untested.

Without a doubt, Singapore is the easiest place for that kid to test his assumptions. Most people speak English. Expats are well treated. Housing is comfortable. Still, moving to Singapore put 9,700 miles between me and everything I knew.

"Travel is fatal to prejudice, bigotry, and narrow-mindedness," Mark Twain wrote.[2] He's not wrong. In Singapore, I learned Chinese, poorly. I joined a blues band, a little less poorly. I found Singapore's artists and rebels. I explored its alleys, picked up its patois, and dove deep into its colorful underbelly. And I left the island as much as work would allow—to Thailand, Vietnam, Cambodia, Malaysia, China, Indonesia, and Mongolia. Living in hovels, eating on dirt floors, accompanied only by a journal and a sketchbook, I climbed to the tops of temples and watched the sun sink behind vistas unchanged over centuries. I saw both the beauty and the ravages of poverty. I learned to hate tourism from the position of the privileged tourist.

In the 1990s, before the Trans-Siberian railroad* became so tourist-heavy as to price anyone else out, it shuttled Mongolian traders across Siberia, men who trekked from Ulaanbaatar to Moscow every two weeks, dressed in the furs they planned to sell.

It also had a reputation for lawlessness. Splitting the bottom two bunks of my four-berth cabin on that train was an elderly Russian couple. During the seven-day journey, they rarely left their beds. They subsisted on dried fish they bought through the window at every station stop and a single pornographic magazine they shared with each other. He'd lie on his bunk and read the articles while she made tea from the samovar at the end of the carriage. Then he'd pass it to her. She'd read it, pass it back to him, and he'd start over.

I slept in the upper right-hand bunk, above her. To my left lay a massive Russian soldier. The way he glared at the three of us when he first boarded, I was convinced neither I nor my belongings would survive the trip.

Only three other tourists made the journey across Siberia. The second night, the four of us ate together in the train's single dining car. My roommate and his boisterous crew of Russian military sat at the other end. Drinks appeared at our table, aimed at the two female tourists. Soon, eight of us crammed into a booth meant for four. Vodka flowed, and cards came out. Between our American-accented Russian and their

---

* Although they are often collectively referred to as the "Trans-Siberian railway," the railway system encompasses three main routes. The original Trans-Siberian railway connects Moscow to Vladivostok. The Trans-Manchurian dips into China's northeastern provinces. Finally, the Trans-Mongolian—which is the one I took—makes a southward turn just east of Lake Baikal, connecting through Ulaanbaatar, and ending in Beijing.

Russian-accented English, we taught each other the games we knew until after the rest of the train had gone to bed.

The Trans-Siberian traveled through dodgy parts of Russia. My roommate—and new spades opponent—made sure I and my backpack survived.

The year in Singapore confirmed what I'd suspected—whether I became a linguist in Papua New Guinea, a medical missionary in China, or friends with a card-playing Russian soldier, the moving sidewalk would be soul-crushingly fatal for me. Over sautéed silkworm larvae, fermented mare's milk, and kerosene lamps, I had met wanderers. I had met people who'd stepped off the anodyne paths their families had charted for them. My friends at home, companions on the moving sidewalk headed toward safe retirement, looked nothing like these wanderers with their dirty feet, these nomads who carried little with them besides a guitar.

I knew my why lay elsewhere.

YOU'D THINK THAT REALIZATION would have changed my life, and toward the end of my contract with Ngee Ann, I thought it might. But I am not a brave man.

On a humid, sweltering day—because Singapore only has humid, sweltering days—I rode the subway east, from Ngee Ann to the Immigration and Checkpoints Authority building on Kallang Road, in the center of the island.

I was going to apply for permanent residency, to keep 9,700 miles between me and medical school.

As the subway train slid through Singapore's granite bedrock, my resolve faltered. Nine thousand seven hundred miles is a lot of miles. Was I going to be a teacher forever? Was I really going to move to a country where almost no one looked, spoke, or thought like me? It had already become clear that Adele and I weren't working out.

I convinced myself instead that I wouldn't apply. All I wanted from the Immigration and Checkpoints Authority was information.

I forced myself not to flee the subway train. Dover. Buona Vista. Commonwealth. Prerecorded voices announced the station names in four languages.

Every time ten beeps heralded the subway's closing doors, I willed myself into my seat. What would my mother say if I never came back? This isn't how you treat your family! You don't move ten thousand miles away. You don't dip your toes anywhere near these waters.

Queenstown. Tiong Bahru. Tajong Pagar.

I could have turned around, but I loathed the prospect of flying back to Dallas, back to the maroon medical school halls. Sure, Singapore was hot. Sure, I sweated constantly. But I loved the country. I loved my life. I didn't want the year to end.

Raffles Place. City Hall. Bugis. Finally, Lavender.

I rode the escalator up into the Singaporean heat. "Just questions," I reassured myself. "No decisions." What would it take to keep 9,700 miles between me and medical school? Would I even be eligible? What tests would I have to pass?

Out of the underground, I raised my eyes to that bright white building on Kallang Road. I paced at the subway entrance. I circled the canal the building stood next to, once, twice, like Joshua at Jericho's walls. I stared at the building's doors. I walked up to them.

Then I chickened out, turned around, and went home.

Sometimes, the things we don't do matter most.

Chapter 6

Security is mostly a superstition. It does not exist in nature, nor do the children of men as a whole experience it. Avoiding danger is no safer in the long run than outright exposure. Life is either a daring adventure, or nothing.

—HELEN KELLER

FIFTEEN YEARS AGO, THE emergency room in Bonaire's Fundashon Mariadal Hospital was just that—a room. Six years after Singapore, on another island in the opposite hemisphere, I tried to escape medicine again.

"Would you mind very much dropping your pants?" She looked tired. Her supervising doctor had already gone home that Friday night. Everything about the nurse exuded fatigue. Her voice, her hair, her face. The whites she wore had been dulled by myriads like me. She'd seen my kind before.

A swipe of alcohol, the sharp affront of two needles. "Ativan," she said, "and dexamethasone."

Earlier that day, I'd dislocated my shoulder in a scuba diving accident. My humeral head—the top part of the bone in my upper arm—sat on my chest, radiating a colicky pain through-out my body. She hadn't offered me any pain relief—maybe she wasn't allowed to without a doctor's order—only a steroid and something for the anxiety I definitely didn't feel.

She called the doctor, but it seemed like the doctor didn't want to come in. She called the ambulance driver instead—could he pull my arm into place? He was out on a run in the hospital's single ambulance, so we waited. The pain spread. Her annoyance did too.

The driver was an absolute beast: gargantuan, muscular, and kind. But here's the thing. When you dislocate your shoulder, all the muscles surrounding it seize, their spasms locking the shoulder in place. Strong as he may have been, that physiology was stronger. He pulled, tugged, puffed, yanked. It hurt.

The two of them then turned me prone, attached a ten-kilogram weight to my right wrist, and let my arm dangle. They hoped the gentle pull of the weight would relax the spastic rotator cuff muscles.

It didn't.

When she finally showed up, the doctor's clothes betrayed her Friday night: a glittery purple top, black pants, and high heeled, open-toed shoes. And also, the authority to administer a narcotic. Thank God.

Her manicured nails dug semilunar grooves into my right bicep. She threw my arm over her shoulder like rope, turned her back, and pulled.

"It looks like we're going to have to operate," she said.

"I'm sorry, what?"

"We've tried everything we can. Surgery is the only way to get your arm back in place. But we have a problem. There's only one surgeon between us and Curaçao, and I need to see which island he's on."

Even today, Google returns more hits for surgeonfish than for surgeons in Bonaire. Most surgical disease gets referred to Curaçao, Aruba, or Holland, or it waits for a visiting surgeon.

In 2004, the visiting surgeon was a wiry, diminutive man who strode into the emergency room in an aloha shirt, a pair of blue flip-flops, and shorts that revealed more of his upper thighs than I was prepared for. He untied the weight from my wrist, flipped me on my back, kicked off his right sandal, jammed his bare foot into my armpit, grabbed my wrist, and *pulled*.

And my shoulder snapped back.

Instantly, the pain vanished. I stopped sweating. I could breathe again. Surgery averted.

For a bit. The shoulder is one of the body's least stable joints. Unlike other joints, it moves in every direction, a feat it achieves by keeping the arm bone separated from the socket itself. The humeral head floats free, held to the thorax by the rotator cuff muscles and a few cartilaginous bumpers. Under normal circumstances, your arm can move out of the joint by as much as an inch in any direction.

Freak scuba diving accidents aren't normal circumstances, and the post-relocation MRI showed a tear in one of those cartilaginous bumpers. Turns out, I'd need surgery after all.

STUDIES DISAGREE ON THIS. For the type of lesion I had—a superior labrum anterior-posterior, or SLAP, tear—many authors now advocate conservative management with surgery only in select instances or when conservative management has failed.[1]

But I agreed to surgery because I wanted it to fix both my

shoulder and my career. The man they wheeled into the operating suite six months after Bonaire was not the same man who left Singapore six years earlier.

By the time I went under anesthesia, I'd spent almost half a decade training to be good at something I cared painfully little about.

So far, I've talked about the moving sidewalk as if I didn't have a choice but to take it. That's not fair. I could always have left. I *should* always have left. I'd just never given myself permission to do so. I was too scared to make the decisions I needed to make, preferring instead to wait for miraculous exits—so that I could then not take them.

This impulse—wanting to quit without actually quitting—led me to a specialty I aligned with about as well as a vegan does with a barbecue pit.

I didn't want to write this book because I did things the right way. Instead, I wanted to write it because I made just about every wrong decision a person can make on the road to his why, and because I hope that my stumblings might encourage you to choose more wisely than I did.

WHEN I SLID INTO medical school after my father's death, I made a Faustian bargain: I'd do this thing I never wanted to do only if it got me into missions work in Asia. I may never become a missionary linguist, but at least I could become a missionary doctor.

Back then, people got into missionary doctoring—we now use the more respectable term "global health"—through internal medicine. They treated infectious diseases, especially HIV/ AIDS, tuberculosis, or malaria. I figured I could do the same.

Two internal medicine rotations later, I knew I couldn't. During the first rotation, my team worked under the charge of an attending hematologist. Fascinated by all things blood—and explicitly *not* fascinated by all things *not* blood—our attending decided one Saturday that, instead of seeing our patients in person, she'd have us card flip.

Card-flip rounds are common. Around a conference table, the care team runs the patient panel, detailing any events since the last time they met, reviewing data we each carried on index cards tucked into our lab coat pockets. Card-flip rounds are supposed to be fast, a pit stop before getting back to the work of actual patient care.

These rounds lasted eight hours.

Eight hours, in a windowless room, engaging in exactly zero patient care. Every lab result became a lecture. Our attending hematologist adored the spur cell, a small, spiculated red blood cell sometimes present in patients with liver disease. She spent two hours on it. And I knew that there was *nothing* in internal medicine that could generate as much passion in me as that hematologic urchin did in her.

WITHIN A WEEK OF the start of my second medicine rotation, Ms. Garcia actively tried to die. I saw it happen. I saw the young woman's breathing turn agonal—gasping, slow, and irregular. I saw her eyes diverge until they pointed at opposite sides of the ceiling.

My intern called a code blue, summoning a team with specific expertise in life-threatening events. Until they got there, though, he was in charge. I'd never seen so much fear in a doctor's face. He saw the obvious—Ms. Garcia's symptoms weren't subtle—and he knew he was out of his depth.

So, he retreated to the familiar, to what his attendings had taught him to do. He talked. He taught.

Ms. Garcia to his left, the window to his right, he decided this was the best time to lecture his medical students. His measured, staccato oration wouldn't help Ms. Garcia's breathing, but he didn't know how to do that anyway. He knew how to teach, to dissect a problem, to create a comprehensive differential diagnosis, and to talk through solutions. In the real-world morass of fear, loss of control, and a patient trying to die, he found his balm in facts.

In 1978, Samuel Shem published *The House of God*, a semiautobiographical novel about becoming a doctor in Boston. There are thirteen rules in the House of God. Most are deeply cynical—Rule 13: "The delivery of medical care is to do as much nothing as possible"[2]—but there's one I still repeat to myself in any crisis.

Rule 3: "At a cardiac arrest, the first procedure is to take your own pulse." No patient is well served by a doctor undergoing her own catastrophe. Panic helps neither the doctor nor her patient.

My intern broke Rule 3. He panicked.

Until Dr. Lampe poked his head through the door.

"Need any help?"

Dr. Lampe was a different sort of medicine intern. Unlike my intern, Dr. Lampe wasn't fresh out of medical school. He'd already had a year of training. He started as a surgical intern, but, after that first year, he realized it wasn't for him. He jumped ship, starting over with a second internship in internal medicine. Lampe had a wisdom it would take me another decade to understand: in jumping ship, he refused to compound an initial mistake—choosing a specialty he didn't like—with the mistake of sticking with it.

I'm *really* good at sticking with things. It's the ethos of Work. It's what my people do.

The year of surgical training had given Dr. Lampe a knack for cutting through the chaos. He didn't talk. He didn't construct differential diagnoses.

He fixed Ms. Garcia. Within minutes, she had a large intravenous line in her groin and an oxygen mask on her face. Before the code team arrived, Dr. Lampe had started resuscitation.

I wanted to be like Dr. Lampe.

I SPENT THE NEXT two years systematically ruling out every specialty after internal medicine. Some were easier decisions than others. That my future wasn't in obstetrics, even though a lot of obstetricians work in global health, was piercingly clear. The obstetrics department at Parkland Hospital in Dallas, Texas, delivers one out of every 250 babies born in the United States. A baby is born at Parkland once an hour. Every hour. Every day. Every year. People yell. Others bleed. Others scream. No one sleeps.

When we medical students weren't delivering babies or trying to fall asleep perched atop the paper shredder, we spun hundreds of hematocrits, quick tests for anemia. The labor and delivery service at Parkland Hospital in the 1990s didn't seem to trust the laboratory services at Parkland Hospital in the 1990s. Their students were their lab.

Unfortunately, the wonder of bringing a new life into the world couldn't outshine the sounds, the smells, and the fatigue of obstetrics.

Like obstetrics, pediatrics presents its practitioners perfect opportunities for work in low-resource countries. A quarter of the world's population (and fully 40 percent of the continent of Africa) is under the age of fifteen.[3] Neonatal, infant, and under-five mortality are massive drivers of low life expectancy. But I couldn't crowbar scores of congenital syndromes into my brain, nor could I pump myself up enough to face another mucusy nose or croupy cough on the lap of an anxiously aggressive parent.

I proved even less skilled at psychiatry. The dedicated psychiatric emergency room at Parkland followed a decidedly inhumane design. Individual exam rooms—which inexplicably locked from the outside—formed an outer ring. At the center of the ER stood a control box, which locked from the inside.

Care teams sat in the control box, behind scratched, bulletproof windows. We wrote notes, tweaked medication dosages, and researched symptom constellations. Between the control box and the exam rooms lay the Moat, a linoleum expanse to which patients were relegated.

Eight hours a day, we sat in the central core, separated from the Other by plexiglass and locked doors. We only braved the Moat for one-on-one patient exams behind more locked doors.

I met so many Jesuses that month, so many people sexually obsessed with their neighbors, so many who inched their chairs closer to the single window to hear messages from other planes.

I met paraphiliacs, schizophrenics, sociopaths. I saw faces chiseled by years fighting deep-seated personality disorders, pariahs chained to linoleum because their brains terrified us. I saw the Other, safely shielded by bulletproof glass. They stayed in the Moat, because their Otherness terrified us.

I also met the socially acceptable psychiatric patients, those whose pathology didn't scare us. With the psychiatry of the acceptable, rehabilitation was the goal. Depressed, anxious, and dysthymic patients got air-conditioned, white-and-gray psychiatric offices, mass-produced art prints, and rooms that didn't lock. They weren't in the Moat. In them, we saw us. There, but for the grace of God, we went. Thank that same God, though, that we hadn't been made a Moat patient.

I CAME PERILOUSLY CLOSE to choosing a specialty for the right reasons.

Cataracts cause colossal worldwide disability, and fixing them takes literal minutes. As organs go, the eye is also among the most mesmerizing. So many things happen within two pyramidal holes in your skull—micrometer movements, under the control of minuscule muscles powered by a complex netting of nerves. An intricate lacrimal system keeps these two sensitive organs from drying out, because parts of them get no blood flow whatsoever. Rightly so: imagine how different the world would look if blood vessels crossed your pupil.

Cells that see only red or green or blue pepper a gossamer membrane across the back of the eye, sharing pointillist space with other cells that don't see color at all, only light. They're arrayed optimally, held in place by a viscous yet somehow transparent jelly.

These two miraculous little organs work in concert with each other and with the brain, resolving a river of information into three-dimensional sight, all while ignoring your nose.

I had high hopes on the plane back to Singapore for a month-long rotation in ophthalmology. If it went well, my career was set.

It didn't, and it wasn't.

A few years earlier, stuffed alongside thirteen medical students into a fourteen-person van in Matamoros, during a profoundly colonialist mission trip—where medical students barely out of college practiced their diagnostic skills on people who lived atop a literal garbage dump, offering no treatment except Flintstones vitamins and short courses of aspirin—Dr. Stephen Lacey told us how to choose a specialty. "Don't focus," the gastroenterologist said, "on the cool parts of a job. Every specialty has them, but they're cool because they're rare. They don't sustain a career. Instead, pick the specialty whose bread and butter you don't hate."

I don't totally agree with Dr. Lacey. Life isn't about figuring out which boredom is the least boring. But there is wisdom in his advice: while every job has its ups and downs, we spend most of our time between the two, mired in the mundanity of the day-to-day. Even at the center of your purpose, some Mondays are just Mondays. No career has enough dramatic highs to overcome a hatred of the everyday.

I disliked ophthalmology's everyday. The cool parts were undeniably fascinating, but the quotidian made me numb. I saw a banal, orthodox future, an assembly line of cataracts stretching out for decades. Pop one out, replace it with a precisely tuned plastic prosthesis, wash your hands. Pop. Replace. Wash. Pop. Replace. Wash.

It doesn't help that we surgeons can be an arrogant bunch. In Singapore, I met abrasive, abusive surgeons, chief among them the head of ophthalmology at the hospital hosting me. This man epitomized the old guard, a species of sexist surgeon whose extinction can't happen soon enough. He took puerile pleasure, for example, in the fact that the word *implant* can be used for both the plastic lens he put into patients' eyes and silicone imbeds other surgeons slid into breasts. More than once, he quizzed his all-female nursing staff about his personal breast taxonomy. There were, he said, three types: papayas, oranges, and bee stings.

And he yelled. He threw instruments—at the wall, at the ground, at people. He said positive things only about himself, reserving vitriol for patients, nurses, medical students, and his residents. He impressed himself with his own abilities, like how he could, in a single movement, doff his gloves and slingshot them into the trash. To be fair, he was really great at it. I never saw him miss.

That skill validated his surgical prowess, he claimed. Gloves midair, he'd remind us, "If I ever can't do this, I will retire. You can't be as good as I am without perfect hand-eye coordination."

He was good. Really good.

I never wanted to be him.

Chapter 7

"Do you find yourself sort of secretly hoping that civilization collapses," Melissa said, *"just so that something will happen?"*

—EMILY ST. JOHN MANDEL

IN SUCCESSION, EVERY SPECIALTY toppled, shot down like plastic ducks at a state fair. And of course they did. They didn't have a chance because I'd never bought into the whole medicine thing in the first place.

The problem wasn't the specialties themselves. It wasn't that ophthalmology was too boring or that kids were too croupy. It was the fact that I wasn't willing to admit that my path wasn't my why.

Instead, I became a perfectionist in the search for specialties. I refused to settle for anything besides the Platonic ideal, the single specialty that would make me immensely happy. That specialty didn't exist because, in a field I'd never wanted to be a part of anyway, *nothing* would have made me immensely happy.

Purpose, meaning, and contentment exist when why is at

the center, and when we construct our paths to lead to it. Not the other way around.

Instead, I flipped everything. I subjugated why to the path I was already on, forgetting that I'd never wanted to be on it in the first place. By flipping the hierarchy and elevating how over why, I made satisfaction impossible. The right choice would have been to recognize this and to do what Dr. Lampe had done. Jump ship. Start over.

But I was too scared.

Too scared of what my family would say, of whether I'd go broke, of what I'd be leaving behind, of what things I might regret. So, instead, from among the slurry of specialties, I had to force one to work.

Medicine won. The allure of safety, security, cachet, privilege, income, and the chance to own a Jaguar won. Living in Asia faded. Hudson Taylor faded. The thrill of the life I had daydreamed receded behind an inertial veil.

I began to believe that everything would just get better if I stuck it out. Medicine is a respectable profession, I reminded myself. Quit dreaming, Mark. Grow up.

My God, I hate how easy it is to flip hierarchies, to idolize safety, security, money, privilege, cachet, and the chance to own a Jaguar. How easy it is to exalt path over purpose.

Instead of asking, "What am I best suited for?" I convinced myself to ask, "How can I best suit myself to the path I'm already on?" Instead of reconsidering the path itself because it didn't fit my purpose, I discarded the parts of my purpose that didn't fit the path.

With the addled wisdom of a mind deprived of sleep for four years, I decided that the best way for me to choose a specialty, the best way for me to survive the path I was on, was to find one that would allow me to work as little as possible, and to make as much money as possible, so that I could do all the other things in my life I wanted to do. Like linguistics. Or playing guitar for Petra.

That specialty was otolaryngology. We got precious little exposure to ear, nose, and throat in medical school, but I'd heard good things. ENTs were supposed to be the happiest surgeons. They'd figured out the lifestyle issue, balancing a clinical practice with an active external life. They were the nicest surgeons, too, the most well-rounded. They tailored how much surgery they did. They could choose to treat conditions—tonsillitis, allergies, reflux, or ear infections, for example—that responded to simple medications, or they could perform some of the most complex surgeries done in any operating room.

An otolaryngologist might one day swing half a patient's face to the side to remove a tumor growing from the bottom of her skull and then reconstruct the defect with tissue from her leg. The next day, he might spend hours with his eyes pressed against a microscope, removing the smallest bone in the body and replacing it with a metallic piston.

The eight inches of the human body between the top of the lungs and the bottom of the brain carry a complex, intersecting, and crucial labyrinth of anatomy. It's tiger country in there. One misstep and the ENT renders a patient permanently unable to move his tongue. Another false move, and the patient is permanently hoarse.

It's a fascinating specialty. And the rumors I'd heard fit my criteria: it paid well, got the doctors home at a decent hour, and gave them weekends off. It was exactly what someone who wanted as little to do with medicine as possible needed.

Chapter 8

If a system is corrupt, then the people who adhere to the system, and are incentivized by that system, are not criminals. They are victims. The system itself must be tried.

—DAVE CHAPPELLE

On OCTOBER 4, 1984, a college student from Vermont was admitted to the New York Hospital in Manhattan with a flu-like illness. She was dead within twenty-four hours. Her death certificate listed the cause as cardiac arrest.

The real story is bit more complicated.

During her hospital stay, Libby Zion was under the care of Luise Weinstein, an intern three months out of medical school, and Gregg Stone, a second-year resident. In addition to Libby, Weinstein and Stone were responsible for a panel of forty other patients that overnight shift, on a different floor of the hospital. Weinstein had already been on call for at least seventeen hours by the time she started treating Libby.

She served as the primary caregiver. After Stone gave his instructions for Libby's care, he tried to catch a few hours of sleep. He remained available by pager as necessary.[1] The senior doctor of record, Raymond Sherman, was on call from home. Although he was consulted, he did not see Libby that night.

When Libby first showed up at the hospital, Weinstein and Stone diagnosed her as having a viral illness "with hysterical symptoms." They prescribed meperidine, a synthetic opiate used for moderate-to-severe pain.

Over the course of the evening, Libby became increasingly agitated. Weinstein initially restrained her chemically with haloperidol, an antipsychotic drug used for agitation, then prescribed physical restraints.

Because the meperidine interacted with an antidepressant Libby was already on, the patient's temperature rose. By 6:30 a.m. the next day, it had broken 107 degrees Fahrenheit. Weinstein initiated emergency measures, but Libby died from the heart attack she suffered that morning.

WHAT HAPPENED AFTERWARDS CHANGED the face of American medicine.

Libby's father, Sidney Zion, was a New York lawyer and a one-time writer for the *New York Times*. Her mother, Elsa Zion, was a publishing executive.

Neither believed the death certificate or the hospital's official story. They were convinced that their daughter didn't die from an overreaction to a viral illness, but from a deeper, systemic issue in American medicine. In Sidney Zion's words, "They gave her a drug that was destined to kill her, then ignored her except to tie her down like a dog."[2]

Libby's parents blamed understaffed hospitals and overworked doctors for her death. "You don't need kindergarten to know that a resident working a 36-hour shift is in no condition to make any kind of judgment call, forget about life-and-death," Libby's father wrote in an op-ed column.[3]

Her parents pushed for criminal murder charges against the physicians, which—unusually—the Manhattan district attorney allowed. Although the grand jury failed to indict either Weinstein or Stone for murder, they did charge them with thirty-eight counts of negligence and incompetence.

Five years later, the New York State Board for Professional Medical Conduct, which had been tasked with investigating these thirty-eight counts, unanimously acquitted Weinstein and Stone of all charges. The New York State Board of Regents reversed the medical board's verdict but decided that "censure and reprimand" would be sufficient punishment. The New York State Supreme Court would ultimately clear the doctors of formal censure.

At the concurrent civil trial, the defense insisted that Libby's death was "tragic but unavoidable." However, Stone, Weinstein, and Sherman were found guilty of negligence and were ordered to pay $750,000 (reduced to $375,000) to the Zion family.[4] Both Weinstein and Stone still practice medicine in New York City. The ripple effects of their case continue to be felt nationwide.

After the grand jury indictment, the state board formed a commission of experts to evaluate Sidney Zion's claims of lethal systemic issues in medical training. The New York State Ad Hoc Advisory Committee on Emergency Services (also known as the Bell Commission, after its chair, Bertrand Bell) would end up recommending that residents work no more than eighty hours a week, and no more than twenty-four hours consecutively.[5]

In 1989, New York State adopted these recommendations,

along with a requirement that attending physicians be in-hospital at all times.

Change did not come immediately, however. The Bell Commission's recommendations were nonbinding. The Accreditation Council for Graduate Medical Education, which regulates American residency programs, was under no obligation to comply with them, and they didn't for a long time.

In 1990, six years after Libby Zion's death, the ACGME set rules similar to the Bell Commission's recommendations—an eighty-hour-maximum workweek, overnight call no more frequently than every third day, and at least one twenty-four-hour period off every seven days. But they only applied these rules to internal medicine, preventive medicine, dermatology, and ophthalmology departments.

It wasn't a sweeping transformation—only 25 percent of the over thirty-one thousand residents in the nation are in these four specialties.[6] For three-quarters of medical trainees, nothing changed.

I STARTED MY OTOLARYNGOLOGY residency in 2001, at the same hospital where Libby Zion died seventeen years previously. The Bell Commission's recommendations floated in the ether—amorphous, ignored, whispered asides. We knew they existed, but most surgical subspecialties, mine included, had escaped the ACGME's attention.

We took pride in this. We were surgeons. We were tougher than those other doctors, what with their sleep schedules and call schedules and work-hour limits. We didn't need those. We thrived in fire. We welcomed hardship. We boasted about our one-hundred-twenty-hour workweeks.

Our days followed an insistent rhythm. Mine started at 1:30 a.m. with a taxi ride to the hospital for "pre-rounds," a solo, middle-of-the-night visit to every one of the forty to eighty patients I covered on my service.

On pre-rounds, I gathered vital signs, lab results, wound and dressing status, and any salient overnight events, which I would present to the rest of the team when they arrived at five. No patient got more than a couple of minutes' attention because the operating room started by seven o'clock. Evening rounds began at six o'clock if we were lucky, nine if we weren't. Then it was home for a few hours of sleep before the cycle began again.

Every second or third day, I took overnight call. On these nights, an on-call intern took responsibility for multiple services. The senior resident spent the night either in the operating room or asleep in the call room.

There were only two rules for overnight call: don't let patients die, and don't wake up the senior resident.

Long days, interminable call nights, and sleep deprivation led to short fuses. And alcohol. And gallows humor. And more alcohol. And a palpable sense of just barely keeping it together.

We were proud of what we did, though. We *were* the front lines. Not a lot of people, we told ourselves, could work like this. Not a lot of people could make split-second, life-and-death decisions on two hours of sleep, sustained by Twinkies and packaged cafeteria cheese cubes.

We may have known how ludicrous this was. We may have known that it was the same hubris that Sidney Zion decried more than a decade earlier. But the hustled nights stoked our pride. We were the infantry, one phone to each ear and multiple pagers nagging from our hips. We were the only thing standing between our patients and their otherwise certain demise.

THINGS CHANGED IN 2003. Petitions to the Occupational Safety and Health Administration led to congressional proposals to regulate work hours for residents in all specialties, nationwide. The ACGME balked. Instead of ceding its authority to the government, it decided to self-police.

Overnight, rules that had once applied to only four specialties bound the rest of us, except without any additional personnel. The work we used to do in one hundred twenty hours had to be done in eighty, and the change happened in a day. Resistance was swift and fierce. It still is.

Large fines accompanied any breach, which forced this resistance into hiding. Attending surgeons couldn't explicitly tell us to overstay our hours, but they could wink at it. "I'm *supposed* to tell you to go home now, but Dr. D has a great case this morning that no one else can cover."

Were you a real surgeon, these suggestions implied, or would you go home to sleep?

This was the exact dilemma I found myself facing in the spring of 2004. Honestly, the choice wasn't hard. I'd just come off a mercifully quiet overnight shift, and Dr. D's case genuinely was good. I wouldn't have missed it.

But I should have.

The ACGME conducted an unannounced compliance check two days later. I did my best to cover for my breach: I told the ACGME's enforcers that I'd gotten adequate sleep the night before; that I only watched the case; that I was responsible for absolutely no medical decision-making.

But they would have none of it. I'd broken the law, and my residency program had let me. The program was to blame, and the ACGME would have to fine them $50,000.

A week later, lathering our hands over a scrub sink, my chairman asked what happened.

"I had to cover Dr. D's case," I told him.

He paused.

"Looks like I'm suing you for $50,000."

He rinsed off and walked into the operating room.

IT'LL COME AS NO surprise, then, that I hated ENT. My residency program was aggressively unkind, my chairman had threatened to sue me, and the specialty hadn't made good on its promise of letting me do all the things I wanted to do outside of medicine. I wasn't playing music or becoming a linguist.

I hadn't escaped the moving sidewalk. Far from it. I'd been cheated.

Kaylin Ratner, a researcher out of Cornell University, defines *derailment* as "perceived changes in identity and self-direction." In her research, subjects who experienced life derailment had difficulty reconciling how their current lives had unfolded with the lives they grew up thinking they would have. These subjects, she wrote in 2019, "do not easily identify with their former self."[7]

Because of the cognitive dissonance that derailment causes, its psychological impacts can be felt for years. Anthony Burrow and his colleagues, also out of Cornell, found that individuals who experience derailment face a significantly higher risk of depression up to eighteen months after the derailing event—a risk that exists *even if* the participant feels like the derailment actually changed their lives for the better.[8]

That resonates. By the time I chose ENT, nothing looked familiar anymore. I couldn't identify with my former self. I had forced his dreams down, locked them out. The dreams could look in, but they'd lost the right to speak. Their voices had become so painful that, for my own safety, I had to silence them.

Where I had once wanted to be Hudson Taylor, medical missionary, I had become Mark Shrime, nose picker.

Don't get me wrong. Although there's a lot amiss with the American medical system, countless people find meaning and satisfaction in it. For many of my medical colleagues, clinical practice *is* their why.

If it had been mine, I might have been more inclined simply to lie to the regulators that day. I wasn't. I resented my specialty, the hospital I trained in, my chairman, and medical practice itself.

For sure, I convinced myself that telling the regulators the truth was an act of integrity and honor, but in reality, it was just another attempt to escape the moving sidewalk without having to make the choice to leave it myself. If I could convince the regulators to shut down the whole residency program, then I could leave without having to quit.

At the start of Dr. Ratner's paper on derailment, she quotes the author Andrew Solomon:

> In June 1994, I began to be constantly bored. My first novel had recently been published in England, and yet its favorable reception did little for me. I read the reviews

indifferently and felt tired all the time. In July, back home in downtown New York, I found myself burdened by phone calls, social events, conversation. The subway proved intolerable. In August, I started to feel numb. I didn't care about work, family, or friends. My writing slowed, then stopped. My usually headstrong libido evaporated. All this made me feel that I was losing myself.

I felt all those things: bored, angry, disillusioned. Every pager chirp triggered visceral fury. I snapped at colleagues, nurses, friends. But I couldn't muster the courage to leave. Better, I subconsciously decided, to burn the whole thing down.

RESIDENCY IS OBJECTIVELY HARD. A recent study in *Biological Psychiatry* found that, over the course of their first year, residents age six times faster than normal adults.[9] It's not just that we're tired and stressed. It's that we're actively driving ourselves toward an early death.

As a result, we turn to clichés to numb the derailment—food, alcohol, drugs, gambling, and sex. A survey of 417 British doctors—who, incidentally, are limited to only fifty-six-hour workweeks[10]—found that 44 percent of them binge drink and 5 percent meet the criteria for alcohol dependence. One in twelve has a binge-eating disorder and one in three experiences strong negative emotions associated with eating. Up to 60 percent report a sleep disorder, 70 percent are chronically fatigued, and 12 percent suffer with moderate or severe insomnia.[11]

Thursday mornings at the Columbia/Cornell otolaryngology program are reserved for Grand Rounds. Lectures, conferences, and board exam preparation sessions all happen on those mornings.

Attending physicians with the misfortune of having to operate on Thursday mornings are left uncovered by the residents, cursed with writing their own orders and wheeling their own patients to the recovery room.

I forget who first suggested that we go gambling in Atlantic City on a Wednesday night, but whoever it was met no resistance. If we could get out of work by six, we could catch a bus from Manhattan to Atlantic City and be back in time for Grand Rounds the next morning.

The on-call residents covered the rest of us, herding us out of the hospital in time for the bus. We gambled and drank and sang obnoxiously to piped casino music all night in Atlantic City.

At two in the morning, standing on a cold, unlit New Jersey beach, throwing jetsam back into the black water, we had the philosophical conversations only possible among chronically sleep-deprived friends. We were honest with each other. We admitted how much we actually hated residency. We broke the thrall medicine held us under. For one night, boorish and drunk, we were free.

We caught an early bus back to Manhattan, showered in the call rooms, changed into fresh sets of scrubs, and made it to Grand Rounds with no one the wiser.

I peppered my residency with escapes like this. None as monumental as overnight escapades in Atlantic City, but escapes nonetheless. While everyone hates residency, some of us hate it more.

Because medicine hadn't kept its end of the Faustian bargain, my escape attempts took on an unhealthy urgency. It strikes me just how toxic I must have appeared to my friends. It's a miracle—and a testament to them—that we're still friends.

MY CHAIRMAN AND I aren't. It may seem weird that he threatened to sue me, but he wielded a familiar cudgel. Every year, 7 percent of doctors are sued—surgeons even more frequently—and, by the time they reach the age of sixty-five, almost every physician will have faced at least one lawsuit.[12] Although 80 percent of suits never result in a payout, when payouts are awarded, they're huge: $500,000 on average for a settlement, and over $1 million for suits that go before a jury.[13]

A third of suits are for "failure to diagnose," forcing physicians into playing defense. Four out of five physicians admit to ordering unnecessary tests because of a fear of liability,[14] and 74 percent of doctors unnecessarily refer their patients to specialists just to cover themselves.

David Hemenway, a Harvard economist, calls medicine a *credence good*.[15] Most things we buy, according to Hemenway, are easy. Cheddar cheese, for example. There's nothing risky about cheddar cheese. We see its price, and we know how much we like it. To Hemenway, cheddar is a *search good*; we know both sides of the equation—price and outcome—before we buy.

For other things, we know the price, but we can't predict our satisfaction until after we've experienced them. A new car and an unfamiliar bottle of wine are such *experience goods* in Hemenway's taxonomy.

Medical treatment—and especially surgery—is neither. As a patient, you know *nothing* about what you're about to buy. You don't know the price until you get the bill, and you can't predict how well treatment will work before you've undergone it.

All you can do is believe that your surgeon did the right thing (hence, *credence*). We literally put you to sleep, do stuff inside your body, and sew you back up. You have no choice but to take your surgeon's word that all went well.

And here's the kicker: you can't even know an operation's quality *after* you've received it. Observing the result isn't enough. The most ham-fisted surgeon can still remove a tumor, and sometimes even the most elegant surgeons don't succeed.

Results aren't necessarily an indicator of a surgeon's skill. Either you have the credence that your surgeon did her best or you don't.

The evidence suggests that whether you believe your surgeon is based on whether you like her. A landmark study of medical litigants, physicians who'd been sued, and physicians who hadn't been sued found a striking patient-doctor disconnect.[16] Litigants described their doctors as neither open nor honest, but 80 percent of defendant doctors said their relationships with patients *were* honest.*

Consistently, studies show that patients sue their doctors because they feel devalued, deserted, and misunderstood, and not necessarily because they've had complications.[17] Patients sue because they feel that, without suing, they'll never get a satisfactory explanation or compensation.[18] Communication breakdown, not a doctor's skill, is the primary cause of malpractice suits.[19]

On the other hand, doctors think patients sue because they

---

* Notably, however, 95 percent of physicians who were *not* sued felt that they entered into honest relationships with patients.

want to find someone to blame. Because over half of medical lawsuits find that the complication couldn't have been avoided, doctors end up feeling like they're being blamed for something they couldn't have controlled in the first place.[20]

Lawsuits place a heavy burden on both patients and providers. Although a payout occurs every forty-three minutes in the US,[21] the toll of lawsuits far outstrips their monetary effect. A quarter of physicians describe being sued as one of the worst experiences of their lives.[22] They detail an irrevocable break in the doctor-patient relationship: they no longer trust their patients, even those who didn't sue them.

Suits also expose a provider's dormant self-doubt. They isolate providers; they break marriages and families.

Surgeons who have been sued are more likely to report depression, burnout, exhaustion, detachment, and suicidality.[23] This sets up a vicious cycle: burnout leads to more mistakes[24] and, consequently, more lawsuits.[25]

Litigation haunts every aspect of medical culture, creating a schism between doctors and their patients. As Albert Wu of Johns Hopkins University says, "If people are consistently beaten up when there's a bad outcome, you create a climate in which no one talks about anything."[26]

There are second-order effects too. Doctors funnel much of their salaries into medical malpractice insurance. An obstetrician in New York State can pay over $200,000 per year just to cover malpractice.[27]

AND PATIENTS FEEL IT.

Despite scads of research on the effects of lawsuits on physicians, I could find little evidence for what happens to patients after a lawsuit. To explore this more, I spoke with members of ProPublica's patient safety community group, all of whom had filed lawsuits (both successful and not).

I've changed their names and identifying details, but they all gave me remarkably consistent stories.*

They told me they felt trapped in an authoritarian system: "We experience medical oppression. Healthcare providers are free to maim and kill...because attorneys will not litigate. [We] need to rein in these psycho doctors. They are doing more damage than good and lying through their teeth," said Jason, a plaintiff whose suit was ultimately unsuccessful.

Victoria, who settled her lawsuit, talked about "unscrupulous healthcare workers who pharmaceutically rape their elder patients by penetrating them with a hypodermic needle... against their will and without their consent."

Others threatened violent retaliation on their physicians. Maria, another plaintiff, warned, "Eventually, you will see vigilante activities against doctors. When a doctor has, on multiple occasions, shown reckless disregard toward his patients, eventually someone will snap."

They spoke of their frustration at an apparent lack of consequences. Brad, who was left disabled after a medical error, said, "I could not get justice. But the doctors and hospitals that did this to me are still moving on. These medical professionals we blindly put our faith in sleep well at night, with no regard for the debilitating impact on our everyday life and our future. I live in a constant state of fear, anxiety, anger, and depression."

---

* All quotes were either made in a public forum or explicit permission was obtained for their inclusion.

Alexander, another litigant, reported the same depression, anger, and fear, all of which extended to his family: "My twenty-five-year marriage ended. My family has never been the same. We lost our home and our friends. My eldest son, who is now twenty-eight, can't even discuss sickness. I am hyper-vigilant; my startle reflex is far too active."

Patients find themselves unable to trust a health system in which they, simultaneously, feel trapped. "It makes finding doctors harder. I'm not a medical professional so my opinions are devalued by doctors," Alan said.

Woody, a nurse himself, told me, "It leaves a bit of an ache in my heart. I still do not trust *any* doctors. Because of my role as a nurse manager, I have been in too many closed-door meetings in which alcoholic physicians are covered up because they generate money for the hospital, or verbally abusive physicians are left undisciplined because they provide a steady supply of admissions to the hospital. I feel more afraid than ever. Health-care has become only about money. I do not think I could work with doctors. I do not think that would be safe."

Almost everyone I talked to leveled accusations of record tampering and alterations after the adverse event. Jason wrote, "My records are full of errors and half-truths."

It's a distrust that seeps into the rest of patients' lives. Sean told me, "If a person discounts or disregards my experience, in any way, the relationship ends there. It's not the adverse event itself, but the defensive position taken against patients afterward, that upsets me."

Michelle Mello, a lawyer and health policy researcher who has studied the effects of medical malpractice on the industry, told me that she suspects that patients may have difficulty disentangling their feelings about the lawsuit from their under-lying unresolved anger about both being injured and having uncompensated injury costs. On average, litigants pay up to 40 percent of their awards back to their lawyers, and most report emotional, financial, and relational trauma.[28]

STEEPED AS MEDICINE IS in litigation, is it any wonder that my chairman threatened to sue? Although he never made good on that threat, it was the only enforcement mechanism he knew.

Physicians enter medicine out of an idealized desire to help people. I did. I'm sure my chairman did too. Instead, we find ourselves mired in a culture of animosity—between patients and physicians, between physicians and their colleagues, and between the healthcare system and everyone else.

The problem, however, isn't physicians, and it isn't patients. It is the asymmetric, inequitable system we're trapped by. Unwittingly, by threatening to sue me, my chairman forced me to start thinking seriously about this system. He set off a chain of disillusionments that would eventually lead me to solve for why.

I only needed one more.

Chapter 9

The struggles we endure today will be the "good old days" we laugh about tomorrow.

—AARON LAURITSEN

I MET SAMUEL DURING my first year as a full-time clinician.

Despite a combative chairman and a specialty I'd never really learned to love, I finished residency in otolaryngology.

A subset of otolaryngologists focuses on cancers of the head and neck. I encountered these surgeons late in my residency training, and, as much as I may have disliked general ENT, I liked what they did. Head and neck cancer is fascinating, the surgeries even more so. And I adored my patients.

I signed up for a fellowship in Toronto to train in head and neck cancer surgery. The Liberian car crash that started this book happened at the end of that fellowship.

I loved the surgeries I did in Toronto, loved the people I worked with, and grew to love that Canadian city, despite lacerating winds that shot up University Avenue from Lake Ontario.

I wrote my fellowship essay about the opportunity that cancer gives its practitioners to stand at the interface between doctor and priest. We get to flex technical muscles and also to sit with patients and their families at the single most potent juncture in their lives.

I met patients in Toronto whose stories stay with me. Angelo had an early-stage cancer. He was exactly as old as my father would have been had he still been alive. His tumor should easily have gone away with appropriate treatment, except it didn't.

I watched as the realization came over him and his family that we wouldn't be able to beat this. I watched his grace as he accepted the inevitable outcome. His steadfast love for his daughter never wavered. His sly attempts to set her up with eligible single men in the hospital didn't either.

As we finally discharged Angelo from active care and into hospice, I watched him thank everyone for working as hard as they did, for pouring energy into his life.

He poured his energy into ours.

THREE YEARS, A LIBERIAN car crash, and a second fellowship after I met Angelo, I moved to Boston, where I began work as a cancer surgeon at a large hospital in the southern part of the city. That's where I met Samuel. He had been referred to me by his primary care doctor, who had noticed an asymmetry in his tonsils. One was larger than the other.

A little bit of anatomy is important here: Each of us has two tonsils, perched above our tongue, one on each side. The tonsils form part of the lymphatic system; they're one component of a ring of infection-fighting tissue inside our mouth, nose, and throat. Because they're only a small part of the lymphatic system, however, removing tonsils has never been shown to increase the risk of infection. In fact, for some rare immune conditions, removing them is the only treatment.[1]

Of course, any surgery is painful and comes with a risk of complications. For tonsillectomies, one of the most common complications is mouth hemorrhage—which is as terrifying as it sounds.

Surgeons therefore take tonsils out only when it's indicated, and asymmetric enlargement is among the clearest indications we have. Up to 5 percent of patients with tonsillar asymmetry hide a cancer in the larger tonsil.[2],* Although cancer often comes with other symptoms—pain, difficulty swallowing, weight loss, and fevers—and although it's associated with things like being older, using tobacco and alcohol, or having a history of human papillomavirus infection, none of these is required.

Samuel was young, a nonsmoker. He rarely consumed alcohol. He had no other symptoms. His primary care provider had found the large tonsil incidentally, on a routine checkup.

After he told me his story, I examined his head and neck. I put a flexible endoscope down his nose to see if I could find any other enlarged masses. I asked about fevers and weight loss. I felt for enlarged lymph nodes in his neck, in his armpits, near his elbows, and in his groin. Everything looked and felt normal.

Nobody wants to hear the c-word. Once the specter of cancer enters the conversation, nothing else matters. For good reason: cancer is a terrifying diagnosis; I lost my father to it and watched Angelo and other incredible patients succumb to it.

---

* I'd be remiss not to quote other studies, however, that find no association between isolated asymmetric tonsillar enlargement and cancer. See, for example, Fikret Cinar, "Significance of Asymptomatic Tonsil Asymmetry," *Otolaryngology—Head and Neck Surgery* 131, no. 1 (2004): 101–3.

Surgical oncologists know that if we're going to mention cancer, we need to be prepared for the conversation that follows.

Samuel's enlarged tonsil wasn't subtle, however. Even if I didn't find other signs of cancer, I couldn't rule it out in his case. The specter had to enter the conversation. His tonsil was large and the only way to be sure it didn't harbor a malignancy was to take it out.

Our conversation took the better part of an hour, much to the chagrin of the waiting room. We discussed his two options: we could get his tonsils out, or, because there was a 95 percent chance this *wasn't* cancer, we could watch and wait.

WE HUMANS AREN'T GOOD at probabilities. We overestimate the chance of uncommon things, especially when those uncommon things are bad,[3] and we underestimate the chance of the common.

Objectively, a 5 percent cancer risk is small. But if it were my tonsils, I'd take those offending things out. That's 5 percentage points too many. With cancer, I want certainty.

When it comes to surgery, however, others take a different tack. Mouth hemorrhage sounds awful. Plus, surgery hurts. An equally reasonable response to asymmetric tonsils would be to leave them in. A 95 percent chance of not having cancer might be good enough. These patients are more surgery-averse than they are cancer-averse. When probabilities are in their favor, they steer away from the knife.

This was the scenario I presented Samuel. Small chance of cancer, which we could turn into a near-certain yes or no if he had surgery. But also, an equally small chance of mouth hemorrhage—and a 100 percent chance of pain—if he had surgery.

He needed to think about it. A week later, his parents, his brother, and his partner all perched on chairs in my examining room. His tonsils hadn't changed. He still had no other symptoms.

"How sure are you it's cancer?" he asked.

About 5 percent.

"Have you done cases like this before?"

Hundreds.

"What would you do if you were me?"

That question is really hard to answer.

On the one hand, decision paralysis is a real thing. Sorting through possibilities and uncertainties, especially under the specter of cancer, can be stupefying. Sometimes, we just want someone else to make the decision for us.

On the other hand, we jealously protect our autonomy. We don't actually want a doctor to force us to do anything. So, instead of having the doctor tell us what to do, we ask him what he'd do in our shoes.

A friend of mine makes critical choices with a coin flip— not because she's cavalier, but because she thinks the moment of greatest clarity occurs in the split second after the coin leaves her hand. If she pays attention, she catches a fleeting hope about how the coin will land. Her psyche, she claims, knows the best choice, and the coin flip surfaces that intuition without any rationalizations.

Samuel's question is akin to that coin flip. When I answer it for patients, I often see imperceptible changes in their faces. Sometimes, a wave of relief washes over. Yes, that's what they wanted to do. It's comforting to know they were making the "right" decision.

Sometimes, their jaws tighten slightly. They wanted to do something else. They hoped I'd say anything different.

I told Samuel what I'd do: I'd have my tonsils out. His face didn't change. No wave of relief, no jaw tightening. He just nodded and walked out.

I never saw Samuel or his family again. We scheduled a second follow-up appointment, but he never showed up.

"Want a surgery you don't need? How about cancer?" he wrote in a Yelp review.

A two-paragraph screed followed, detailing his evidence that my only goal—like all doctors—was "lining his pockets." Thank God, he wrote, he had gone to seek a second opinion at a different hospital in the city. Thank God a "real doctor" told him he had no need to worry. Thank God the doctor could tell, just by looking at him, that he definitely didn't have cancer.

Renegade doctors like me, he claimed, needed to be corralled. We couldn't be left unchecked, psychopathically wheedling our patients into surgeries they didn't need, scaring them with words like *cancer*, just so we could strike it rich.

Although I was angry about that review for months, my intention here isn't to malign Samuel. It's to highlight the final disillusionment that pushed me off my moving sidewalk and onto the road to why.

MEDICINE IS A SERVICE industry, and, over the decades I've been a doctor, it's become more industry than service. Nowhere is this more evident than in the exaltation of patient satisfaction scores.

The use of "objective" patient satisfaction measures has skyrocketed since I started in medicine, driven in part by a single company. Press Ganey, which has cornered the market on patient satisfaction surveys, partners with nearly half of all hospitals in the United States.[4] Multiple studies have shown weak (and sometimes zero) correlation between their scores and objective patient outcomes,[5] while other studies have demonstrated racial[6] and gender[7] biases in how patients respond to their surveys. But none of this has stopped them. They're a lumbering behemoth between you and your doctor.

Press Ganey's ubiquitous satisfaction scores are only supposed to be used to benchmark hospitals against themselves. Obviously, they're not. Hospitals flaunt good patient satisfaction scores. Bad scores cause administrative insomnia, because bad scores mean fewer dollars.

Hospitals use these satisfaction scores to compete for market share. They also use them to pit individual departments against each other.[8] Quarterly reports used to appear in our inboxes, rife with color-coded comparisons with our colleagues: yellow for average, green for above, and red for insomnia-inducing.

The Centers for Medicare and Medicaid Services, or CMS, has also gotten into the patient satisfaction game.[9] This is even more problematic: because CMS drives medical reimbursement, where they go, all of American medicine goes. They currently withhold 1 percent of Medicare payments for hospital-based purchasing, 30 percent of which is tied to patient satisfaction scores.[10] Satisfaction-bound reimbursement is only expected to increase.

The problem is, the science of satisfaction is complex. Reliably reducing a subjective feeling to an objective, color-coded number is impossible, because human emotion is complicated.

But color-coded numbers allow split-second comparisons, so they've become a singular goal of the patient encounter.

This is dicey talk. I don't mean to imply that the patient experience should be devalued. On the contrary, no patient should ever feel disrespected, unmoored, or unheard by their doctor. No patient should encounter rudeness from me, the nurses I work with, or anyone else in the hospital. Like any service industry, we should care deeply about how good our service is and how satisfied our customers are when they leave our offices.

Ours, however, is a different sort of service industry—no one expects the halibut at their favorite restaurant to save their life or to diagnose their enlarged tonsil—which means doctors sometimes have to say things their patients don't want to hear. Sometimes they have to address the potential cancer in an enlarged tonsil. Sometimes they have to scare us, to make us uncomfortable, to put us through things they wouldn't want to go through themselves. They wouldn't be doing their jobs otherwise.

This isn't to say that doctors shouldn't learn to be more communicative, that we shouldn't work to make our patients as comfortable as possible as we're telling them difficult things. This isn't to say that we can't do better.

But it is to say that the exaltation of poorly validated, color-coded satisfaction scores to the position they now hold is specious.

And it's deadly. In 2012, Joshua Fenton and his colleagues at the UC Davis Medical Center published a scathing investigation of patient satisfaction in the *Archives of Internal Medicine*.[11] Using eight years of data from CMS's satisfaction survey—and over fifty thousand patient encounters—they measured the association between color-coded satisfaction scores and health-related outcomes. Of all the satisfaction domains measured by CMS, they chose the one that drives most lawsuits: communication between patients and their providers.

In their rigorously controlled analysis, the authors found that patients reporting the highest satisfaction scores were counterintuitively more likely to be admitted to the hospital in the next year, more likely to face higher healthcare costs, and more likely to spend more on prescription drugs.

And more likely to die. The most satisfied patients were 26 percent more likely to be dead over the next seven years than other patients.

It's possible that this is a spurious finding: maybe the most satisfied patients were also the sickest ones who therefore had the most to gain from a medical encounter. To make sure this wasn't the case, the authors redid the analysis with only the healthiest patients—and the correlation got stronger, not weaker. Healthier patients who scored high on patient satisfaction measures were 44 percent more likely to die over the next seven years than less satisfied patients.

And that's the fundamental problem with viewing medicine as a service industry. If Fenton and his colleagues had found no mortality difference, then color-coded satisfaction comparisons would be annoying but necessary. If hospitals could provide the same level of medical outcomes, if they could keep their patients alive at the same rate no matter the satisfaction scores, then pursuing color-coded satisfaction as a primary goal would be absolutely correct.

But that's not what's happening. A robust study using the

best-validated survey of patient satisfaction finds the exact opposite. The highest color-coded numbers correlate with the worst mortality.

This sits very poorly with me. It runs counter to the oath we doctors swear to uphold. We do harm by focusing on these satisfaction scores. A groundswell of resistance to these scores exists, but it hasn't reached the people who need to hear it most: the administrators.

AND THEY ARE LEGION. Between 1975 and 2010, the physician workforce grew at about the same rate that the population did in the United States. Over the same period, the healthcare administrator workforce grew 3,200 percent.[12]

According to the United States Bureau of Labor Statistics, there are sixteen nondoctor workers for every doctor. Six of those sixteen have clinical roles—nurses, physician assistants, or other allied health professionals.

That leaves ten other people without clinical responsibilities: for every one doctor, there are *ten* administrative employees with no patient contact.[13] An administrator workforce that's ten times the size of the physician workforce it's supposed to support will, without doubt, create significant bloat in healthcare costs.

It could be argued that mushrooming healthcare costs are due to the ever more complex care that patients demand, but the science doesn't support this. Between 2002 and 2012, for example, the total number of days Americans spent getting inpatient care went *down* 12 percent.

What administrators focus on instead is color-coded comparisons and profit. They impose layers on suffocating layers between patients and their doctors. In 2016, researchers directly tracked the movements of fifty-seven clinicians across a broad range of specialties. For every hour a doctor spent in patient care, she spent *two* hours doing administrative work.[14]

We'd never allow that in any other career. Imagine a twenty-minute sale taking an entire hour because the employee has to document the conversation, word for word, in case someone wants to sue seven years later.

We wouldn't allow it in any other career, but we celebrate it in medicine.

A similar motion-tracking study of 142 family physicians showed them working twelve-hour days, every day. Then, *after* that twelve-hour day, they spent another ninety minutes just finishing off the paperwork they had left over from clinic.

Literally half of the twelve hours weren't spent with their patients either. Instead, these doctors spent six hours with the electronic health records their hospitals (and the US government) require them to use. Forty-four percent of those interactions were documentation, billing, coding, and system security. Managing their inbox required an additional 25 percent of the doctors' time. Only 32 percent of the hours that physicians spent with health records related to clinical care.[15]

To put this in perspective, interacting with patients—the thing we want our doctors to do—is a full-time, eight-hour-a-day job. The health system extracts an additional five and a half hours *per day* from doctors, just to manage all the administrative things no one else is doing. Including those ten administrators.

And all this is in the service of profit.

It isn't clear that extra documentation helps patients in any way. It is clear, however, that it helps charge capture. Hospitals shift administrative requirements to physicians not because they improve patient care but because they bring in more money.

Which puts doctors in a bind. They are, correctly, punished for poor outcomes. It's a risk they know they bear.

But, instead of improving outcomes, they must focus on the things that improve their employers' bottom line: documenting minutiae, churning through an unrelenting torrent of patients seven minutes at a time, and ordering enough tests to justify the defensive medicine they're forced to practice.

And they can't stop, because each doctor-patient interaction supports the salaries of sixteen people. Each interaction bolsters the stability of the administrator phalanx, while doing little for either the patient or the physician.

It's an unwinnable bargain. The risk of bad outcomes falls on doctors, but the benefit of good outcomes accrues to hospital ledgers. Patients become throughput and doctors the assembly line.

IF IT'S AS BAD as I'm saying, though, why do people keep becoming doctors? Why don't we revolt?

Because most of us went into medicine to answer a deeper calling. Danielle Ofri, a physician at Bellevue Hospital in New York City, has written that, despite the corporatization of medical care, "most clinicians remain committed to the ethics that brought them into the field in the first place.... An overwhelming majority [of doctors and nurses] do the right thing for their patients, even at a high personal cost."[16]

This ethic supports a miasma of competing priorities,

misaligned incentives, threats of litigation, and antagonistic interpersonal relationships. "If doctors and nurses clocked out when their paid hours were finished," she writes, "the effect on patients would be calamitous. Doctors and nurses know this, which is why they don't shirk. The system knows it, too, and takes advantage."

We won't even shirk for the right reasons. A survey of physicians and midlevel providers in Philadelphia found that, although 95 percent believed that working while sick put others at risk, 83 percent still did it at least once in the prior year. The majority of these respondents cited fear of ostracism by colleagues as a driving factor in their decision.[17] European physicians do the same: between 70 and 86 percent of physicians in a survey from Italy, Sweden, Norway, and Iceland reported regularly coming into work while ill.[18]

We take a similarly hard-line approach to mental health. A strong stigma toward healthcare providers with mental illness thrives "as a result of the culture of medicine and medical training, perceptions of physicians and their colleagues, and expectations and responses of health care systems and organizations," according to a 2017 paper by Jean Wallace, from the University of Calgary.[19]

Doctors are one and a half times more likely to be dissatisfied with their work-life balance than the rest of the nation, and almost twice as likely as their nonmedical friends to suffer from emotional exhaustion, depersonalization, and overall burnout.[20]

Almost four hundred physicians will kill themselves this year, twice the rate of the national average.[21] The physician suicide rate exceeds that of combat veterans.[22] Suicide is the second-most common cause of death among medical students, second only to accidents.[23]

It's for this reason that over half of physicians would not recommend medicine to someone just graduating from college.[24]

THERE'S SO MUCH MORE I could tell you, so many more things to indict the American medical system. I could write entire chapters on the mutual distrust patients and doctors can have for each other, on the nefarious effect of science denialism and of TV doctors who are more often wrong than right,[25] or on the fact that physicians are incentivized by volume—paid to do more, not better.

But that's not the point. Being a doctor still carries with it some of the cachet, income, privilege, prestige, and job security it did in the past. It's still a steady road to success, and for many, it's still their why.

My point, instead, is to describe the thousand cuts a life outside of why inflicts, the life I found myself living before the Liberian car crash. It's to detail the walls that closed in on me, and the distress I felt in realizing that the Faustian bargain had failed.

It's to describe what I escaped when I solved for why.

Chapter 10

—◆—

His dream must have seemed so close that he could hardly fail to grasp it. He did not know that it was already behind him, somewhere back in that vast obscurity beyond the city, where the dark fields of the republic rolled on under the night.

Gatsby believed in the green light, the orgastic future that year by year recedes before us. It eluded us then, but that's no matter—to-morrow we will run faster, stretch out our arms farther.

—F. SCOTT FITZGERALD

I N COLLEGE, I WORKED as a waiter at Burger King.

It only happened in a few test markets in the mid-1990s, this waiter thing. Princeton, New Jersey, was one of them. Late in the fall, a sign appeared on the window of the Burger King on Nassau Street, just north of campus. Red Bauhaus letters on cheap white paper promised eight dollars an hour.

I'd just been turned down for a job at a tutoring company. Not that I could blame them; I bombed the interview.

No small feat: all I had to do to get the tutoring job was

to teach a small group of fellow applicants anything I wanted. Literally anything. The guy who got the job taught us how to make paper airplanes.

Me? I wanted people to learn how to pronounce the word *fire* in the most metal way possible. If you want to sound like a *real* rock star, I told my fellow interviewees, you had to pronounce the word with two syllables.

That, honestly, was the sum total of my lesson plan: write *fy-ur* on the white board. Wait for jaws to drop.

Rejected, I got myself a Whopper and a job as a waiter at Burger King.

HERE'S HOW IT WORKED.

"Hi! Welcome to Burger King!" I'd chirp as you walked through greasy glass doors.

More often than not, you'd stop short. Burger King has greeters? Since when? And why was I so cheery? And also, would I get in the way of you and your Whopper?

It turns out, yes. I would.

I'd herd you toward an open table. You could refuse—you could just walk up to the counter yourself instead, but most people didn't. Most people were too shocked.

After I settled you onto your grim plastic bench, I'd hand you the menu, which was also the disposable tray liner.

"I'll give you a moment to decide," I'd say, motioning at the yellow, red, and brown pictures on unctuous paper.

When I came back, it was with your free appetizer, a bag of popcorn from the carnival popper propped against the far wall.

"What can I get you today?"

I'd write your order down on the greasy short-order slip I

kept tucked into the dirty blue apron I picked up from behind the restaurant counter every shift.

And then, as you watched, I'd take my place in line behind all the regular Burger King customers and await my turn to place your order. While we both waited for the ding of a hotel call bell affixed to the counter—signaling that I could walk your order from the cash registers back to your table—I'd mop the floor and clean the bathrooms.

Needless to say, waiters didn't last long at Burger King.

BECAUSE THE BULK OF my professional life has been in medicine, I'm most familiar with its dissatisfactions. However, professional dissatisfaction isn't limited to the white coat. It's rampant in our culture and especially ubiquitous among those of us who haven't solved for why.

As I mentioned in the last chapter, medicine is a service industry. Sure, doctors go through a lot of schooling. Sure, you're more likely to die at the hands of a physician than at the hands of a Burger King waiter. And sure, you—or your insurance—will pay much more for our services than you would for your Whopper.

At its core, however, clinical practice is a service. Unsurprisingly, then, the dissatisfaction that I found in medicine exists in many other service industries. A friend of mine works as a line cook at a restaurant in a big American city, for example. He talks about restaurants the way I talk about medicine. He loves making people happy, celebrating major events, and cooking the food people like.

And he also hates service industry culture. He hates the dehumanization that accompanies it, in the same way that I hate the dehumanization that accompanies clinical practice in the United States.

All this is to say, work is hard, and my story isn't unique. Doctors don't have a monopoly on dissatisfaction and burnout. Charles Duhigg, author of *The Power of Habit*, has written in the *New York Times Magazine* about his fifteenth grad school reunion at Harvard Business School. As incoming business school students, he writes, "what really excited us was our good luck. A Harvard MBA seemed like a winning lottery ticket and—if those self-satisfied portraits that lined the hallways were any indication—a lifetime of deeply meaningful work."[1]

Duhigg and his fellow grad students desired the same lifetime of deeply meaningful work that I'd been pursuing—vainly, so far—since I had resigned myself to not being Hudson Taylor.

But just like an MD doesn't confer on its holder a lifetime of deeply meaningful work, the Harvard MBA disappointed Duhigg's friends as well. "It came as a bit of a shock," he continues, "to learn how many of my former classmates weren't overjoyed by their professional lives—in fact, they were miserable."

He gave a few extreme examples—of corporate politics, of backstabbing colleagues, and of companies stolen from under noses—but dramatic stories of dissatisfaction are few. Most chairmen don't threaten to sue their residents.

Instead, he writes, "most of us were living relatively normal, basically content lives. But even among my more sanguine of classmates, there was a lingering sense of professional disappointment.... They complained of jobs that were unfulfilling, tedious or just plain bad."[2]

* * *

THIS LINGERING SENSE OF disappointment is the most insidious danger of life on the moving sidewalk. We face a boring dystopia, a deep-set ennui, and a resignation to them both. I felt it as a doctor, and you may feel it in what you do. Many of us just surrender to it.

Sandeep Jauhar, who wrote *Doctored*, concludes his 250-page screed against the ills of modern medicine with a similar white flag. After asking whether there's "anything more depressing than the manicured patch of lawn in front of the local bank," his denouement is bland resignation.

"Today," he writes, "I am living my life in archetypal roles: often doting father, occasionally reserved husband, at times discouraged doctor.... I will muddle through this."[3]

Jauhar, Duhigg, and I. We're not alone. Most people hate their jobs.

In a 2017 Gallup poll, 85 percent of respondents reported disliking their jobs. Only 15 percent of us find a sense of purpose, passion, or deep connection with our work.[4] The majority of us—63 percent, according to the survey—simply feel nothing about work. We are, to use the words of an accompanying *Forbes* report,[5] "unhappy but not drastically so." We've raised the white flag. We "sleepwalk through [our] days, putting little energy into [our] work."

The remaining quarter of us actively try to sabotage our work. We're so unhappy, we just want to blow it all up. We would jump at the opportunity to tell a regulator we'd overstayed our mandated hours in the subconscious hope that it would bring the whole enterprise down.

I was in that group. You may be too. Or you may be in the 63 percent who just feel blank. No matter: both surrender and sabotage are lethal to a life of purpose—one of them is simply more dramatic.

THE FUNDAMENTAL PROBLEM, HOWEVER, isn't work itself. Work is necessary.

A little over a decade ago, I spent four months unemployed. This was after the Liberian car crash and a return to Toronto for a second fellowship. For the first two weeks, I loved unemployment. I did all the things I'd put off for fifteen years. I slept in. I went out. I cooked. I exercised.

It was amazing. For two weeks, I drank freedom like a shipwrecked man drinks fresh water.

For two weeks.

Then, freedom turned into tedium—instead of going out, cooking, or exercising, I spent hours on my apartment floor, playing Risk with online strangers.

Desperate for something meaningful, I threw myself at the game. I made spreadsheets, optimized army movements, and worked out the probabilities of success with an all-in strategy for Madagascar.

I kept looking for jobs during those four months, only without success. Massachusetts has the highest physician-to-population ratio in the nation,[6] and I was an unknown, a recent graduate of schools in New York and Toronto, with no Boston experience. Employers smelled my desperation.

I applied for any job I could find. Starbucks. Burger King, again. The local bookstore. Restaurants. I scoured the meandering streets of the city, popping my unannounced head into any shop and forcing my résumé on any proprietor who didn't immediately kick me out.

This strategy netted a single interview with a now-defunct bookseller. The morning of, I put on my best tie, my best sweater, and my best slacks. The manager ushered me into a tiny interior room, where, surrounded by boxes of unsold books, we sat at a single table, and he asked a single question.

"Why do you want this job?"

I'd prepared for this. Armed with a list of the books I'd read that year, I told him how important good writing was to me, how it soothed and excited and transported, how I couldn't wait to share it with other people.

The truth is, I wanted to work for the bookseller not because I love books (I do) or because I'm transported by skilled writers (I am). I wanted to work for him because, despite optimized Risk probabilities and Malagasy armies, I felt useless.

Work provides us three things: a means of survival, a source of self-determination, and a connection with others.[7] What it doesn't provide is a why. Work is path, not purpose.

Eighty-seven percent of us hate our jobs because work can never meet deeper, existential needs. It cannot give us actual meaning. It may stave off feelings of uselessness, but looking to work for meaning consigns us to the boring dystopia of Duhigg's fifteenth grad school reunion.

THIS IS THE FUNDAMENTAL disconnect I felt in medicine for fifteen years.

I had successfully stuck it out on the path I was on, through years of training I disliked, through a residency fueled by alcohol and Cheez-Its, through aborted attempts to leave the doctoring life, through threatened litigation by supposed mentors, and through months of unemployment—and finally, I landed a job as a doctor in Boston. I made it. The moving sidewalk worked. I found a good career.

More than good. Doctoring is the apotheosis of the American dream, especially for the firstborn son of an immigrant family. On the faculty at a large hospital in a large East Coast city, I found the promise of traditional success.

On the outside, it was perfect. It was what every parent wants for their child.

On the inside, I died.

WHAT ABOUT YOU? ARE you on the moving sidewalk? Are you hemmed in by responsibilities you've inadvertently tripped into while sticking it out on a path that isn't your purpose—mortgages, school payments, parental pressures, spouses, kids, and obligations?

Are you simply enduring life until you can retire? Are you worried that you might not be able to retire? Are you stuck in a job that provides contact with people and a means of survival, but does so at the cost of your soul?

You could—as many people do—just quit it all. You could leave the life you have in a fit of despondency, buy the new car, and move to a different country. You could detonate the path you're on, hoping that, when the pieces land, they'll land in a slightly more tolerable order.

You really could. This gambit works sometimes. A large British study, for example, suggests an eight-to-ten-year increase in happiness with second marriages that's not seen in first marriages.[8]

Or you could resign yourself to the boring dystopia of

Duhigg's class reunion, sleepwalking through your days, putting little energy into your work.

If that sounds depressing, that's because it is. I've lived it.

But bear with me. Read on. I found my way off the moving sidewalk. And on the other side of it lie satisfaction, meaning, and deep fulfillment. On the other side of solving for why lies the life you were called to, the life you deserve.

The way there is going to take grit. It'll take you into failure. It'll throw you headlong into anxiety. It'll pin you to the walls of doubt.

But it'll also revitalize you with wonder, with faith, and with worship.

Solving for why has made all the difference. That's what the rest of this book is about.

Chapter 11

In the space between yes and no, there is a lifetime. It's the difference between the path you walk and one you leave behind; it's the gap between who you thought you could be and who you really are; it's the legroom for the lies you will tell yourself in the future.

—JODI PICOULT

Don't GET A KIDNEY stone in Kyrgyzstan. At least, not on a Saturday.

At three o'clock in the morning on October 13, 2007, I woke to a dull, insistent, colicky left flank pain. It started inconspicuously, a nagging ache that would crescendo, peak, and decrescendo, teasing relief before pummeling my side again. I'd gone to bed the night before with a wicked case of food poisoning, so I moved preemptively to the bathroom.

It wasn't food poisoning.

Kidney stones aren't subtle. Colicky flank pain should have been my first clue, especially when it became so severe that I couldn't sit still. In the textbooks, kidney stone patients writhe in their beds because no position is ever comfortable. I writhed on that bathroom floor for hours, hoping its cold linoleum would quell the spasms in my side.

In retrospect, I had a few risk factors. My brother had kidney stones, as did my father: his cancer had been misdiagnosed as a kidney stone because of this history. I'd been traveling without ready access to clean water, so I was dehydrated, which the prior night's food poisoning didn't help. I'd also compounded the dehydration with a mild diuretic to fend off altitude sickness.

Kidney stones are as easy to treat, however, as they are to diagnose. Unless you're in Kyrgyzstan in 2007.

Painted a clean white with pale blue accents, the Kyrgyz Republic President's Hospital's doors didn't completely close, but its speckled, tan linoleum floors were clean.

My translator brought me there first; we arrived at eleven thirty. Because the Kyrgyz Republic President's urologist only worked until noon on Saturdays, we were immediately sent, on foot, to the nearby public hospital. We were told by the Kyrgyz Republic President's urologist's secretary, "There, maybe, I think, they should be working."

The doors at the Kyrgyz National Republican Hospital didn't seem to close, either, but that's where the similarities ended. The Kyrgyz National Republican Hospital was a dark, dripping, dirty, dire, dank, and desolate place. It felt like the place people go to die.

The on-call urologist saw me, pounded his inconsiderate fists against my back, and sent me for an X-ray he probably didn't need: of all the ways to diagnose a kidney stone, X-rays are the least sensitive.[1]

On the way to radiology, I limped past cinematically squalid inpatient wards. In one, an old woman doubled in prayer at the edge of her bed, lit by a single, naked bulb. In another, a backlit mother and child directed their empty eyes at the wall ahead of them. In a third, a man moaned on a cot while his neighbors studiously looked anywhere else.

And don't get me started on the hospital's bathroom. Middens from past occupants floated in places they shouldn't have. I gave a urine sample in a well-used, barely rinsed baby food jar and a stool sample into a cone of last week's newspaper. Dante once described hell's occupants as "a people smothered in a filth that out of human privies seemed to flow." He could have been writing about the Kyrgyz National Republican Hospital.

Predictably, the X-ray didn't find a kidney stone. The urologist should then have given me pain medicines and hydration before sending me on my way. Most kidney stones pass on their own.

He didn't. He twirled the hairs on his Mephistophelian goatee and dug in.

It was time, he said, to shoot contrast up my urethra because the only cure to my kidney stone was an operation.

I refused.

Reluctantly, he sent me to a private sonographer down the street who quickly located the two offending pebbles in my left kidney. Back at the Kyrgyz National Republican Hospital, the vindicated urologist insisted that—finally!—it was time to cut.

"What did my tests show?" I asked.

"Well, you know," he said. "Tests. They could be one thing today and another thing tomorrow."

I insisted. He gave in: my tests confirmed what the

sonographer had already found. Was I positive I didn't want him to operate?

Defeated, the urologist passed me a prescription written in pencil on Big Chief paper. He ordered intravenous fluid, two herbal medications "for the urine," and, at last, a single injection of pain medication. None of which the hospital stocked.

But if I could buy them myself at the pharmacy across the street, he would welcome me back to the hospital where, for another small fee, he'd happily administer them. On Monday.

My other option, he said, was to hop on my left foot as often and as vigorously as possible—but on the instep only; the outstep just wouldn't do.

The correct treatment for an uncomplicated kidney stone in an otherwise healthy male patient is IV fluids, pain medicine, and tamsulosin, a medication that relaxes the ureters, helping stones leave the kidney. At no point in my trek through the Kyrgyz national health system was I given the correct treatment. I finally got it when I bought my own drugs from a local pharmacist without anyone's prescription ("I'm a doctor" was all she needed to hear).

I got the right treatment because I was privileged: I knew the correct management and had the money to purchase it. No other patient in that derelict hospital could say the same. Through no fault of their own, they were trapped under naked light bulbs, defecating in toilets filled with the excrement of their neighbors, and at the mercy of a system they didn't understand.

These patients had lost the birth lottery. They'd been born into poor families, in countries without the infrastructure to care for them. They'd been born Other, their lives predetermined to suffer under goateed urologists. They were the unlucky ones. They had no choice but to submit to diseases they didn't want and treatments they couldn't reject.

In that Kyrgyz hospital, I caught a fleeting glimpse of what would become my why.

IMAGINE, THE PHILOSOPHER JOHN Rawls wrote in *A Theory of Justice*, that you're tasked with designing the perfect society— but there's a catch. You only get to design behind what he calls a "veil of ignorance." That is, you're not allowed to know what happens to *you*, specifically. You design society before you're born, ignorant of how you'll end up in the birth lottery.

Behind this veil of ignorance, Rawls writes, no one knows "his class position or social status; nor does he know his fortune in the distribution of natural assets and abilities, his intelligence and strength."[2] Small chance you're Warren Buffet, larger chance you're a Kyrgyz kidney stone patient. Small chance you have the intelligence of a Nobel Prize winner, the strength and poise of an Olympic rock climber, the looks of a supermodel. Larger chance you're waiting to die in a forbidding hospital bed.

From behind the veil of ignorance, Rawls asks, what sort of society would you design?

I find his answer remarkably compelling. He proposes that even the most self-interested person would design a society that maximizes fairness and improves the lot of the worst off, because they themselves might be born the worst off. Behind a veil of ignorance, Rawls claims, we all prioritize the Other. The society we currently have—which preferences the already privileged because of some arcane notion that they "earned" it—would never survive the veil of ignorance.

If you can't know whether you'll end up enslaved or some-one who benefits from enslaving others, then a society with slavery becomes a lot less attractive. If you can't know whether you'll have the privilege I brought to the Kyrgyz kidney stone or you'll be at the mercy of a knife-happy urologist, then a soci-ety with the Kyrgyz National Republican Hospital becomes untenable. If you can't know whether you'll be Othered or the one who Others, then racism, sexism, abuse, homophobia, injustice, and an ethos of the Other cannot stand.

It would take me another decade to articulate this into a book, but that Kyrgyz kidney stone planted the first seeds of my purpose. My why—how I would hope to spend the rest of my life—would eventually contradict every ethos I grew up with. It would work to reverse the ethos of the Other, to weaken the worship of exclusionary absolute truths, and to glorify mean-ing over effort.

It would, as much as an imperfect man could, be devoted to justice.

TO FIND THAT WHY, I first had to say yes.

In June, 2005, a friend invited me to a photography exhi-bition in New York City. Scott Harrison, the photographer, would go on to found one of the world's most successful charities, bringing clean drinking water to people in resource-constrained settings. As of this writing, his charity has deliv-ered safe water to over eleven million people in twenty-eight countries.

In 2005, however, Scott was a recently reformed night-club promoter in New York City.[3] He had just spent thirteen months as a photographer with Mercy Ships in Liberia. He wanted to show the folks on his valuable mailing list, which he had curated during years as a promoter, what he'd seen in West Africa.

Still in the middle of residency, I'd only recently decided that I was going to pursue a career in head and neck cancer surgery. There was little my sleep-deprived body wanted to do less than to spend an evening in a dimly lit Soho gallery watching someone talk about a continent I never wanted to work in.

My friend insisted. I said yes.

Scott took the stage. He talked about following patients from their homes to a big white hospital ship, about their trips through the operating room, and about them returning to their families, healed and whole. As the lights went out, he described their transformations. He told stories of doctors working in Monrovia to take tumors off the faces of the Other. He told of health renewed, of sight regained, of faces mended, and of justice restored—all through a surgeon's knife.

AND JUST LIKE THAT, it was time to get off the moving sidewalk. The day after Scott's photo exhibit, I applied to Mercy Ships.

Chapter 12

He who has a why to live for can bear with almost any how.

—VIKTOR FRANKL, PARAPHRASING
FRIEDRICH NIETZCHE

IN 2000, WHILE I agonized over which specialty to choose, a fourteen-year-old boy named Alimou noticed a small lump on his jaw. By the time he got it removed, it weighed seven pounds.

Alimou lives in Guinea, a country of 12.5 million people north and east of Liberia. Although its capital, Conakry, lies on the Atlantic coast, the country subtends an inverted *J*, sweeping above both Liberia and Sierra Leone.

In the deeply forested eastern region of the country, where Alimou is from, proper healthcare can be days away. The national hospital in Conakry is at the end of a forty-eight-hour trip along pockmarked roads only accessible during the dry season.

The government also runs a regional hospital in N'Zérékoré, the city closest to Alimou. However, his access to the hospital was as limited as the services it provided. Surgical patients in every sub-Saharan Africa country in which I've worked face myriad barriers to accessing care—cost, distance, transportation, a lack of providers, a lack of procedures offered by providers, quality, and the fear of being held captive at a hospital until bills get paid.[1]

For Alimou, it made more sense to ignore the jaw tumor than it did to try to get it removed. If you or I were to find a lump on our jaws, we would be in the doctor's chair the next day, and in the operating room within weeks. In fact, in some high-income countries, the maximum time between the first tumor appointment and the first cut of the surgeon's knife is mandated by law.[2]

Not so in Guinea. Over eight years, Alimou's tumor grew large enough to displace his entire jaw and to impede his airway. Unable to chew, he guided pap around the tumor, pushing it far enough back into his throat that it would slide down by itself.

If he lay on his back, the seven-pound intruder obstructed his airway. He hadn't gotten a full night's sleep in years. And the tumor emitted a yellow, sticky smell that forced him to live on the outskirts of his village. "The flies," he told me later, "were my friends."

I met Alimou and his tumor at a mission clinic in N'Zérékoré in 2008, where he joined a line of hopeful hundreds. He'd shown up in response to a radio advertisement put out by Mercy Ships. He hoped we could fix his problem.

We could.

To get his operation, the twenty-two-year-old farmer traveled south, from the forests of eastern Guinea to Monrovia, Liberia. His was the case that finally made me a surgeon.

His was the case that solved for why.

IN WHAT WAS, IN retrospect, another act of desperation, I took a second year off in 2007. After four years of medical school, one year in Singapore, five years of residency, and one year of fellowship—but before the four months of unemployment and the first job in Boston—I'd had enough. Mercy Ships had accepted my application to work with them for six months, and I was going.

Like my mentors ten years prior, no adviser thought this was the right move. They all wanted to know if I'd considered the implications. Did I care how yet another year off would make me look? Was I okay being the doctor who couldn't stick it out, the surgeon too weak to endure surgery? Did I know this would ruin my surgical career?

I wish I could say I was immune to these conversations the second time around. I wasn't. They terrified me. I *hadn't* considered the implications. I *didn't* know how another year off would make me look. All I knew was that I'd hit bottom.

I also didn't know at the time that my mentors were right, that the year off would finally destroy the moving sidewalk of a surgical career. I didn't know I'd end up leaving full-time practice. I just thought I was just taking a second break. I'd be back.

Even at rock bottom, I didn't give myself permission to leave the moving sidewalk. In fact, I took the year off only after making sure clinical practice would be there when I got back. Before I left, I lined up a return to Toronto for a second fellowship in microvascular surgery. One day, I'd need to break the idolatry of safety once for all, but July 1, 2007, wasn't that day.

Lifeline secured, I told my mentors I was leaving.

"I wish I'd done that," one of them told me, sitting in a windowsill in the hallways of the operating department, overlooking a dreary street swathed in slushy Torontonian winter. "Before the kids, before the mortgage, before I had a practice to sustain, I wish I'd taken a year off."

I think about these conversations often. The first ones, the warnings, the preemptive eulogies of my surgical career, weren't the conversations I needed to hear. But I didn't know that then, and my mentors didn't either.

Instead of advice on how to create a successful career in traditional clinical practice, I needed a kick in the pants. Instead of encouraging me to stick it out, I needed someone to push me off the moving sidewalk. I needed someone to see past the security that comes from perseverance. That someone would come, but not yet.

FOR THE FIRST SIX months of my year off, I did leave medicine altogether. Kyrgyz kidney stones aside, those six months were spectacular.

No kidney stones could overshadow the thrill of bargaining with Uighur yak herders in far western China. They couldn't match sunrises over Osh or sunsets that painted Samarkand's blue mosques pink. They couldn't compete with the face-puckering taste of fermented mare's milk in Mongolia, or the cold winds of Everest, or sharing a cramped car with Kazakh mafiosi—or a different car with two constantly drunk Dutch teenagers crushing on their equally drunk, older British travel mate.

Starting in Iceland and ending in New Zealand, I traveled across sixteen countries and two continents, most of it by train. From the soaring, gilded architecture of Saint Petersburg, over the barren steppes of Mongolia, through the dank hallways of a Kyrgyz hospital, to the brilliantly colored geothermal lakes of New Zealand, the first six months off the moving sidewalk were stunning.

The second six were pivotal.

*   *   *

EPIPHANY LOOKS NOTHING LIKE it does in the stories. It comes with no fanfare. There are no trumpets. No angel choruses. No orchestras. No focus-pulled cameras.

I wasn't thrown from a horse on the way to Damascus, nor did an archangel speak the word of God to me. I didn't find enlightenment under a bodhi tree or revelation in two seer stones in a hat.

More importantly—especially for someone like me who enjoys data—epiphany isn't intellectual. It doesn't come from numbers. I could regale you with the disturbing population-level facts behind Alimou's story, but I can't convince you into epiphany.

I could tell you that five billion people around the world can't get surgery when they need it, that only 6 percent of the world's operations happen in low-income countries. I could tell you that eighty-one million people like Alimou are pushed into poverty by the cost of surgical care. And those facts would be as true as they are appalling. But epiphany doesn't live in facts.

Instead, it comes in the quiet, numinous moments that each of us has if we stop to listen. In *The Lazarus Project*, the Bosnian author Aleksandar Hemon writes, "There are moments in life when it is all turned inside out—what is real becomes unreal, what is unreal becomes tangible, and all your levelheaded efforts to keep a tight ontological control are rendered silly and indulgent."[3]

What better way to describe life on the moving sidewalk than that? "Levelheaded efforts to keep a tight ontological control"—over ourselves, our desires, our careers, our lives. Epiphany comes in those numinous moments when the real becomes unreal, and the unreal tangible.

In 2007, a hospital ship called the *Africa Mercy* docked in Monrovia. I walked up its gangplank in January 2008 for a six-month stint as a head and neck cancer surgeon. Mercy Ships, the East Texas–based charity that runs the *Africa Mercy*, takes a unique stance toward the problem of surgery in low-income countries. For four decades, they've provided operations and training from the decks of hospital ships.

Although the details have evolved over forty years, Mercy Ships' hospital ships currently spend about ten months in each country, where they provide between 2,000 and 2,500 surgical procedures for free, where they train dozens of local surgical personnel, where they improve local surgical infrastructure, and where they conduct innovative research.

But again, those are just facts. They're not epiphany.

Epiphany came the first time I walked down the red stairs at the front of the *Africa Mercy*—after fifteen years of post-secondary education, most of which I hated. Stepping off those stairs, onto the third deck, I made a right-hand turn into the maxillofacial and head and neck cancer ward. I saw a dozen Alimous, a dozen patients with head and neck tumors at various stages of recovery. And it finally hit me.

This is what I've been training for fifteen years to do.

THE POET MAYA ANGELOU writes, "Let choice whisper in your ear and love murmur in your heart. Be ready."[4]

Epiphany is rarely grand. It's more often so quiet that we risk missing it. If we aren't ready for it, if we don't listen for it, we too easily get distracted by the drudgery of the moving sidewalk.

Look, there's no way to get off the moving sidewalk without *getting off the moving sidewalk*. Believe me, I tried. I left for

Singapore, chickened out, and came back. I left for Liberia only when I had secured my return to the traditional path of clinical practice. It would take me another three years, and Jacobean wrestling matches with doubt, failure, and anxiety, to leave the moving sidewalk once and for all.

But before I even could, I had to listen.

I had to find those quiet, numinous moments. I had to hear the whispers. I had to ask the questions: Is the moving sidewalk going where I want it to go? Is it taking me where my heart yearns to be?

And the answers came in quietly. I didn't hear them in the winds of work, didn't find them in the waves tossing me from task to task. I heard them at the bottom of a red staircase on a hospital ship in Monrovia.

You won't hear them in the monotony of your moving sidewalk, either, nor will you hear them in the shackles of someone else's plans for you. No. The answers come in the stillness. We hear them when we separate. We hear them when we pause. If only for a little bit.

In *The Heart of Christianity*, the theologian Marcus J. Borg encourages his readers to find what he calls "thin places," where the veil between us and the divine becomes just a bit less opaque.

In the thin places, he writes, "the visible world of our ordinary experience and God, the sacred, the Spirit"[5] intersect. In the thin places, we see that our perceptions of reality, of God, and of our lives are not divine mandates. We see that there's more than just the path we're on. "The veil," Borg writes, "momentarily lifts, and we behold God...all around us and within us."

Thin places are universal. We've all experienced them. We

know their transcendence. We know how it feels to be transported. They aren't the secret purview of mystics. Listening isn't just for the meditators, the bodhisattvas. Thin places are there if we look.

I've found them on Mongolian steppes and at a Mongolian throat singing concert. I've found them working overnight on a particularly thorny research problem and in all-night conversations with close friends. I've found them on silent retreats in central Massachusetts and at the climbing wall at my local gym.

And I found one on a red staircase.

For many traditionally religious people, sacramental cities like Rome, Jerusalem, Mecca, Medina, and Varanasi are thin places, but they don't have to be. My thin places aren't yours. "A thin place," Borg concludes, "is anywhere our hearts are opened...a mediator of the sacred, a means whereby the sacred becomes present to us. A thin place is a means of grace."

Thin places are also ephemeral. We miss them if we aren't paying attention—and we miss them if we force them. They're the faint stars we can see only in our periphery. We can't will our way into the sacred or wrestle ourselves into epiphany. We can't believe hard enough, pray hard enough, meditate hard enough to compel the miraculous.

We can, however, listen. And, while we wait for the thin places, we can cultivate a willingness to be transported when the transport finally arrives and a comfort with the risk that being transported requires.

The veil momentarily lifted for me on the *Africa Mercy*. In that thin place I heard. In that thin place I found why.

Chapter 13

—◦◦—

The opposite of poverty is not wealth; the opposite
of poverty is justice.

—BRYAN STEVENSON

WHEN ANDREW WAS BORN, his mother tried to kill him.

Andrew has albinism, a disease that interferes with the body's natural pigmentation.[1] In some places, people like him are viewed with suspicion or thought to be ghosts. Or they're used as sources of entertainment while simultaneously being spurned in private because they're considered cursed. Sometimes they're seen as so transparent that they could vanish, so they're shunned as devils, sorcerers, or magicians.

Others fear that too much contact with people with albinism* will transmit illness and bad luck. Not true of their body parts, however: fishermen weave their white hair into nets to improve catches. Gold miners use their bones as amulets to increase yield. And having sex with people with albinism is, in

---

* I've chosen to use "people with albinism" instead of the more common "albino" because the latter has taken on derogatory connotations.

some places, thought to cure HIV and AIDS, a belief that has spread the disease widely among folks like Andrew.

In the cosmology of some West African cultures, the human sacrifice of people with albinism was believed to confer strength and power to the king or to quell a rumbling volcano. Ritual amputations and killings of people with albinism were—and still can be—frighteningly common.

There's also a black market for Andrew's organs. The United Nations' Special Representative on Violence against Children has written that "a charm made from their body parts is considered to have magical powers." According to another report from the UN's High Commissioner for Human Rights, "Some even believe that the witchcraft ritual is more powerful if the victim screams during the amputation, so body parts are often cut from live victims, especially children."

IN REALITY, ALBINISM IS genetic, transferable through neither curse nor infection. It confers no special powers, improves no fishing yields, and does not cure HIV. Instead, it reduces the amount of melanin produced in the skin, the hair, and the eyes. Without melanin, a patient's skin and hair take on the ivory color of newly painted hotel walls, and his eyes turn pink. The prevalence of albinism varies fifteenfold across sub-Saharan Africa.[2]

Most people with albinism exhibit marked nystagmus. Their eyes rapidly shuttle side to side, unable to fixate on a single point. To counteract the fluctuations, patients bob their heads in counterbalance. Many are so severely near- or far-sighted as to be considered legally blind.

Although these symptoms diminish quality of life, what

kills patients with albinism in the countries in which I've worked—more than ritual sacrifices and amputations—is cancer. Melanin blocks the cancer-causing effects of ultraviolet light. Without it, Africans with albinism face a skin cancer risk a thousand times higher than the general population does.[3]

These cancers erupt on exposed parts of the body: the hands, the arms, and, especially, the head and neck. Under a tyrannical West African sun, patients like Andrew must encase themselves in suffocating fabric. And when the tumors come—and they invariably do—they bring with them proof that people like Andrew were demons after all.

Andrew got lucky. He survived to adulthood without ritual sacrifice or amputation. He had friends who overlooked the color of his skin and the lurching dance his pink eyes made. He earned his wages playing drums in churches around Monrovia.

Then the tumor started. In the crook of his neck, where his neck met his left shoulder, the skin began to redden and roughen. Soon, the rough patch sprouted mercilessly outward until it became a cobblestoned mass that outgrew its blood supply.

This is common in cancer. Because tumors are a lawless overgrowth of a single cell type, the blood supply they need to sustain themselves doesn't grow as fast as they do. Robbed of oxygen, the central parts of Andrew's tumor started to die.

Andrew's support crumbled as quickly as the fetid insides of his cancer. Because he lived off his drumming, the smell of dead tissue impoverished him. It forced him out of Monrovia and into the slums on its outskirts. His new neighbors demanded that he build his lean-to downwind of theirs.

Born in a country steeped in material poverty, cursed with

eggshell-colored skin, he grew a tumor that—to say nothing of the pain and shortened life expectancy—cemented his social isolation.

IN POVERTY, ANDREW BECAME Other.

A kidney stone in Krygyzstan taught me about justice. Alimou taught me how justice can be invalidated by tumors left to grow unchecked because patients can't access the care they need.

And Andrew taught me about poverty. Our relationship with the Other, whatever it is, is crucial to how we structure our lives. And I believe that the single best way to construct a life of purpose, meaning, and deep contentment—the single fastest path any one of us can take to solving for why—is to turn our hearts toward the poor.

The *only* thing that can save us from our irascibly self-centered existence is to make sure that our existence is in the service of others.

And truly in the service of others. Not in the service of others as a way to glorify ourselves. Not in that counterintuitive pride we can fall into when we find ourselves "doing good."

No. It's in keeping our hearts steadfastly toward the poor.

These aren't original thoughts, obviously. Jesus had them. In the twenty-fifth chapter of the Gospel of Matthew, he separates sheep from goat, sending the former into the kingdom that's been ready for them since the world's foundation.

Why? Because "I was hungry and you fed me, thirsty and you gave me to drink, homeless and you gave me a room."

"What are you talking about?" the mystified sheep ask. "When did we do any of these things?" He responds: "Whenever you did this to the least, to the overlooked, to the ignored, to the poor, to the Other—you did it to me."

For anyone like me, who comes from a Christian tradition, this is a story so familiar as to be toothless. But Christianity is in no way unique in its focus.

Almsgiving is so central to Islam that it is one of its five pillars. In the Mahāvagga, the Buddha gives instructions to his monks to live "for the gain of the many, for the welfare of the many, out of compassion for the world."[4]

And it's not just religion either. Leo Tolstoy flirted with suicide for a year, asking himself "almost every moment whether I should not end matters with a noose or a bullet."[5] During that year, he became consumed by a single question: "Is there any meaning in my life that the inevitable death awaiting me does not destroy?"

There was, he decided. "The sole meaning of life is to serve humanity."

Finally, there's Albert Einstein, who said, "Only a life lived for others is the life worth while."[6]

The safe life is fundamentally a self-centered life. Little is more likely to push us down a Tolstoian spiral than a self-serving life focused on the pursuit of our own happiness, to the exclusion of the Other. The best way to serve humanity, the best way to create Einstein's "life worth while," is to walk with the Other.

In everything you do, turn your heart toward the poor.

I'VE SPENT A CAREER learning about poverty. My research focuses on the ways that accessing healthcare can counterintuitively worsen impoverishment, whether you're in Liberia or in the United States.

And here's what I've learned.

We hold too cramped a definition of poverty. Especially for those of us who come from positions of privilege, poverty feels pecuniary. It's the person on our drive to work sporting a pithy, self-deprecating cardboard placard. It's the mother holding down four jobs to raise her five children. It's the gaunt child we're told we can feed for twelve dollars a month.

It's the person in our church driving a beat-up 2002 Volvo station wagon without air-conditioning that they got for free. It's the man in the downtown shelter, on the street that reeks of micturition and nicotine.

We're narrow-minded when we think about the poor. For sure, monetary deprivation is part of poverty, but its aftershocks are much more subtle. Andrew's poverty was not only monetary; it was also social, and it was spiritual. It isolated. It Othered.

We don't avoid the downtown street because its residents don't have enough money. We avoid it because the people at that homeless shelter feel qualitatively different. Dangerous, even.

We protect ourselves from them and their smells—physically by avoiding them, and existentially through an ethos of the Other. Confronting poverty, then, requires us to take a step back and to turn the spotlight on our understandings of it and reactions to it.

This isn't easy. Most of us want to help. We have an altruistic streak—we see the pictures of the child with a cleft lip, of the orphan with a belly distended from hunger, of the refugees who lost their home—and we react viscerally. We want to *do* something. To change things. To be part of the solution.

If we're not careful, however, we run the risk of making it worse. "We sometimes think that poverty is only being hungry, naked, and homeless," Rashid Rashad wrote. "The poverty of being unwanted, unloved, and uncared for is the greatest poverty."[7]

It's shockingly easy to view the poor as Other, as qualitatively different from us. It's shockingly easy to see their lot as the result of choices *they* made—choices we're sure we wouldn't have made. And in doing so, it's shockingly easy to keep the poor at arm's length. We do our altruistic duty toward the Other and return safely to our lives.

The problem is that poverty's pervasive aftershocks originate not just from a lack of money. They originate from the ethos of the Other. It's easy to see this ethos in Andrew, whose white skin meant he might have been killed for being cursed, but it's harder to see it closer to home, harder still to see it within our own altruistic streak.

Paul Farmer, chair of the Department of Global Health and Social Medicine at Harvard Medical School and founder of Partners In Health, calls poverty "structured evil."[8] This is an off-putting phrase because it implies that those of us outside of poverty—those of us who desperately want to feed the starving child with our twelve dollars—may actually be part of a structure that's keeping the child poor, a structure that's fundamentally evil.

But Farmer is correct. Poverty is at once personal and structural. "Poverty," he continues, "is not some accident of nature but the result of historically given and economically driven forces."

Andrew is an incarnation of these forces. His poverty was

as much individual as it was historically given and economically driven. It was rooted in decisions made by people in privilege long before he was born—in fact, long before even his country was born.

The American Colonization Society—officially the American Society for Colonizing the Free People of Color in the United States—began in New Jersey in 1816. Its goal was to move recently freed victims of American slavery to Liberia, a new American colony on Africa's west coast.

A union of strange bedfellows, the American Colonization Society held competing priorities. Among its constituents were abolitionists like the Quakers who supported "repatriation"— deportation to a country enslaved people had never lived in— because they believed that these enslaved people would never really be given a fair shake in slaveholding America, even after abolition.

There were also the perpetrators of enslavement themselves, for whom the continued presence of free Black people in the United States increased the odds of slave rebellions. Black people, in their eyes, were "promoters of mischief,"[9] so deportation was a way to keep their interests safe.

And then there was Henry Clay, senator from Kentucky, presidential candidate, and Speaker of the House, for whom deportation was "desirable...to drain them off."[10]

Only a quarter of deported people survived, but human sacrifice like this was considered worth it for people like Clay, necessary to secure the future of his homeland for his children. And Andrew's Liberia is a product of these decisions. The back-to-back civil wars that rocked his country from 1989 to 2003 arose from tensions that can be traced directly to these deportations.

The land to which the deported Americans sailed was billed as empty, fertile soil on which they could build their new homeland. Except it wasn't. Local inhabitants resented the invasion of repatriated interlopers, who resented them in return. As the Americo-Liberians resettled in Liberia, they took control of government, and, in an ironic twist of history, the previously enslaved chose to enslave their unwilling hosts.

In 1980, Samuel Doe overthrew the Americo-Liberian-led government. Civil war would erupt nine years later, spilling over into neighboring Sierra Leone, and killing over a quarter of a million people.

So, there's no question that Andrew was poor because he had no money: he lost his job once his tumor appeared. He was also poor because his genetic irregularity made him Other. He was poor because the cancer it caused relegated him to the outskirts of the outskirts.

And he was poor because he was born into a country whose infrastructure had been destroyed by colonialism. He was poor not because of choices he made but because of choices generations before him had made. He was poor because he'd lost the birth lottery that many of us have won. His poverty was historically given and economically driven.

People in poverty do not choose to be in poverty. Andrew's story—and the history it's built on—drives this home: just as we didn't choose to be born where we were born, neither did he. Just as most of us didn't choose to be born with melanin, he didn't ask to be born without it.

Nothing could have changed the lot he drew at birth: a thousandfold higher risk of cancer and a societal structure that viewed him as Other, reinforced in the history of a country shaped by powerful people long since dead. He never consented to any of this, but there he was, with a tumor festering on his left shoulder anyway, driving his neighbors away from him. No amount of skin care, of keeping himself covered, or of staying indoors could have fixed it.

True poverty robs its victims of their seat at the table of humanity. It exists against a backdrop of structural evil. And it survives because of an ethos of the Other.

TURNING OUR HEARTS TOWARD the poor, then, can't just mean dealing with pecuniary poverty. It can't just mean a monthly donation.

It has to mean diving in, walking alongside, breaking down the hegemony, and fighting the ethos of the Other, wherever we find it. It must mean taking a serious look at our own role in perpetuating the structural inequities Dr. Farmer describes. Dealing with poverty means more than volunteering at the soup kitchen on Thanksgiving Day—and more than flying to a ship in West Africa to do surgery.

Poverty challenges us to examine our own assumptions about the poor and forces us to ask whether our fixes are effective. Do they break down the structural context in which Andrew's tumor grew? Or do they primarily exist to assuage our altruistic streak?

If poverty were easily fixable, we'd already have done it. It's not, because fixing it is threatening. We each carry inside us an ethos of the Other. Turning our hearts toward the poor means recognizing that ethos, discarding it, and, in its stead, entering into Andrew's story. The whole of it. The history of it. The religion of it. The ostracism and the tumor and the smells and the wars.

Of all the things I love about my work, I love most the chance it affords to restore to Andrew some humanity. Removing the tumor on his left shoulder—and borrowing his pectoralis muscle and some skin from his thigh to reconstruct the defect—did more than remove a bunch of overgrown cells. It gave back to Andrew his right to look human.

Turning our hearts toward the poor means looking for people like Andrew, people living in shadow. It means meeting the Other, seeing him, walking with him. It means being with him even after the tumor is out. It means acknowledging that there's no quick fix for Andrew's poverty, and working to fix it anyway.

It means making ourselves uncomfortable, letting our charity extend to people who don't look or think like us. It means holding out grace to those who may have made decisions we don't agree with—and who may continue to make them even after we're through.

It means not binding our grace with fine print.

It's easy to send money. It's easy to take out a tumor. Those demand less of us than Andrew's poverty actually does. The specific operations I do aren't my why—they're my how. My why is about restoring justice and breaking the ethos of the Other. It's about Andrew.

Turning your heart toward the poor doesn't have to be on a hospital ship in West Africa. It doesn't have to be grandiose. It doesn't have to be newsworthy. It doesn't have to be what your friends, pastors, rabbis, priests, or colleagues say it should.

It just has to be.

In everything you do, turn your heart toward the poor.

Chapter 14

＊

It comes at its own timing, when I am ready for it—humble, respectful, not expecting it, somehow placing myself lower than it, not above it.

—TIMOTHY GALLWEY

THERE IT WAS. MY why. I'd had the epiphany. I'd articulated what I wanted my life to be about. I'd solved for it.

That should have been it, right?

Well.

Because I had made sure to secure my return to clinical practice before I left for Mercy Ships in 2008, I flew back from Liberia to Toronto and to the planned safety of the anodyne. I completed a second fellowship in microvascular reconstructive surgery, then moved to Boston, where I landed in four months of Risk-fueled unemployment. By January of 2009, I started my first full-time doctoring job in the United States.

A less combative chairman laid out his goals for my job: build a monolithically successful (read: busy) surgical oncology practice, remove head and neck tumors from patients in New England, and reconstruct defects with tissue from other parts of their bodies.

From a fibula, Toronto taught me to create a jaw. From wrist skin, a tongue. From the shoulder blade, a palate. Each piece of tissue was harvested in tandem with its blood supply and transferred to the gap left by the removed tumor. Carefully placed sutures no bigger than a human hair, and even more careful nursing aftercare, usually meant graft survival and a patient with an intact face.

It's thrilling surgery. It's complex, elegant, magnificent. I was good at it.

Also, I didn't like it.

A year into the Boston job, I returned to Mercy Ships for a few weeks. Before I tell you more, though, I have to introduce you to Dr. Gary Parker.

Imagine lashing Jesus and the Buddha together with some wry wit and stuffing them into the six-foot-three-inch body of a missionary surgeon. That's Gary. His why moved him to Africa over thirty years ago, where a temporary stint with Mercy Ships turned into three decades. He met his wife, Susan, on the ship, raised his kids on the ship, and has devoted his entire career to surgical care for the world's forgotten poor.

Operating with Gary is an unparalleled experience. He navigates head and neck anatomy like a New York City cabdriver. The man has seen more Alimous than I ever will.

He's a legend around Mercy Ships. When I arrived to the ship in Liberia, I—no joke—swooned the first time I saw his bald, bearded head. "That's Dr. Parker!" I whispered to the person next to me. "It's him!"

When I returned to the ship the next year, he met me at the top of the gangway, wrapped his lanky arms around me. "My son has come back."

When Gary talks to you, he talks to nobody but you. Four hundred people live on the *Africa Mercy* at any one time, but coffee with Gary is coffee with only Gary. Nothing's off-limits in those coffee conversations: politics to religion to relationships to what approach we'd use in tomorrow's case are all fair.

ONE NIGHT, AFTER A long operation, Gary and I sat in his office for coffee. On the *Africa Mercy*, you meet all sorts of people. You meet caricatures like the dark-haired preacher I grew up with, people whose Christianity necessitates a far-right ethos of the Other, people for whom Jesus is a thing to assent to and a cudgel to maintain hegemony.

And you also meet Gary. Thirty years in Africa have invested in him wisdom. The man's faith impels in him a love toward the Other, a humility toward himself, and an acceptance of imperfection. His why—to restore to his patients their fundamental right to a seat at the table of humanity—bleeds into everyone he meets.

In the middle of our meandering conversation, I asked Gary how he made his life decisions. Three years later, in grad school for decision science, I learned that Gary's answer has a name. It's called the maximax criterion for decision-making under uncertainty.[1]

Or, the Gary Parker Rule.

The Gary Parker Rule is this: when he faces a major decision in his life, Gary looks thirty years into the future at the *best* possible outcome of each of his options. If one of the best possible outcomes makes him think, "Meh," then he *knows* it's not the right choice for him.

Grad school taught me to put numbers to decisions, so

here's a hypothetical example of the Gary Parker Rule. Let's say I'm trying to decide between two career paths, which we'll call A and B:

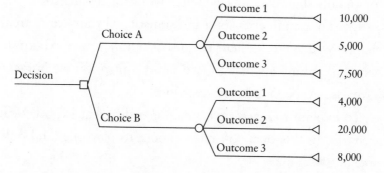

Each path has a set of potential outcomes. In this example, the outcomes have numbers, but these numbers don't (necessarily) have to mean anything. They could mean a salary, or a subjective assessment of your happiness, or the number of ice cream cones you'd get, or how close you are to living your why.

Choosing according to the Gary Parker Rule means finding the best outcome for each career path—10,000 for A and 20,000 for B—and then choosing the best of the best. In this case, because 20,000 is better than 10,000, that's Career B.

It's a risky rule, which is why we rarely use it. Most of us, instead, make decisions using an anti–Gary Parker Rule, or the maximin criterion. Where Gary is optimistic, a maximin decision-maker is a pessimist, focusing instead on making sure the *worst* possible outcome is the least bad it could be. The maximin decision-maker reasons that if things go horribly wrong, at least she comes out ahead. She chooses Career A because its worst outcome—5,000—is better than the worst possible outcome from Career B.

Where Gary asks, "What's the best that can happen?" we

usually ask, "What's the worst?" In the service of safety, the anti–Gary Parker Rule quietly discards joy. By choosing Career A, the maximin decision-maker trades *double* the possible joy for an only slightly more cushioned worst-case scenario.

If the maximin criterion is pessimistic, why are we so trenchantly wedded to it, then? Because it's more secure. Maximin decision-making appeals to two natural instincts we humans have: risk aversion[2] and loss aversion.[3]

To explain risk aversion, imagine a different hypothetical scenario. In this one, you must choose to play one (and only one) of two games.

Game 1 isn't really a game: if you choose it, I hand you $1,000 in cash, no strings attached.

In Game 2, however, you stand to win a lot more. If you choose to play Game 2, you flip a coin. If the coin lands on heads, I hand you $6,000, no strings attached. But if it lands on tails, you pay me $4,000.

Would you play Game 1 and walk away $1,000 richer for sure, or play Game 2, where a simple coin flip decides whether you're $4,000 poorer or $6,000 richer?

If you're like me, you play Game 1. It's a no-brainer: $1,000, no strings attached, without the risk of losing $4,000.

Here's the thing, though: Game 1 and Game 2 are mathematically identical. In both games, you're $1,000 richer on average.

The difference between them comes down to risk. In Game 1, you *know* you're walking away $1,000 richer, while in Game 2, you risk being impoverished, even if, on average, you're still walking away $1,000 richer.

As anti-Garys, we choose certainty over risk.

And we also minimize our losses. With loss aversion, we

ascribe more emotional weight to losing something than we would to gaining the exact same thing.

One last hypothetical to explain loss aversion: imagine that a brilliant scientist has built a happiness meter. With a simple retinal scan, he can quantify exactly how happy you are, on a scale of 0 to 100.

You're one of his test subjects, and on your first retinal scan, the machine reads 62 happiness points. You're mostly happy—not ecstatic, but definitely not depressed.

The next day, prior to getting scanned, you find an envelope in your mailbox containing $500 in cash. Your retinal scan that day will certainly read higher than 62. Every day after that, you find another $500 in your mailbox, and every day, your retinal scan reads high. An extra $15,000 a month goes a long way.

After a month, however, you go to your mailbox, and, unexpectedly, there's no envelope with $500. There's just a note informing you that you will no longer be receiving the daily supplements. Your income drops back to *exactly* what it was before all the envelope nonsense began.

Your retinal scan, however, won't go back to 62. It'll go far lower.

That's because the hurt of losing the $500 per day outstrips the happiness the envelopes provided. That's loss aversion.

We're naturally risk- and loss-averse. We naturally play Game 1.

Solving for why, however, means playing Game 2.

BACK FROM AFRICA, I applied the Gary Parker Rule to my own career. The results weren't what I'd hoped: thirty years as an academic surgical oncologist in Boston meant something like eighty thousand patient visits and ten thousand surgeries. Half of the patients would live, half wouldn't—because that's the nature of head and neck cancer. And I'd retire with a nice house and that Jaguar.

And that was it. That was the end of the moving sidewalk. That's what playing Game 1 led to—and it was everything I'd spent years trying to escape.

The Gary Parker Rule was the final push I needed to get off the sidewalk. "The day came when the risk to remain tight in a bud was more painful than the risk it took to blossom," according to a quote attributed (likely erroneously) to Anaïs Nin. Applying the Gary Parker Rule to my career made it clear: the pain of staying tight in a bud had become too great.

In 2011, three years after I'd met Alimou and Andrew, three years after I could articulate my why, I finally quit my practice—much to the chagrin of the surgeon I had partnered with. Because I knew I wanted to work with patients like Alimou, understanding the decisions they make to seek surgical care and removing the barriers they face, I went back to school for a PhD in decision science, where I wrote my dissertation on the challenges of surgical access in low- and middle-income countries. And I haven't looked back.

I need to make one thing crucially clear: my decision was intensely personal. For my clinical partner, being the best surgeon he could be, delivering the best care he could to his patients, producing the best research he could write, and providing the best life possible for his family—these absolutely drove him.

They didn't drive me, and what drives me doesn't have to drive you.

However, while every why is personal, the things we face in pursuit of it are remarkably similar. Waiting in the space between articulating your why and leaving the moving sidewalk are risk, loss, anxiety, fear, and doubt.

That's why epiphanies are vital to the articulation: there's no reason to face risk and loss except in the service of a purpose that inspires. But while we wait for epiphany, we can start by asking ourselves the Gary Parker question: Does the best possible outcome of our moving sidewalk inspire us?

Because, here's the thing: we can find a thousand quiet, numinous moments; we can have all the epiphanies in the world—and we can still stagnate.

Solving for why means more than just articulating it. It means deciding between Game 1 and Game 2. Between security and purpose.

Chapter 15

―᪥―

To become spring means accepting the risk of winter. To become presence means accepting the risk of absence.

—ANTOINE DE SAINT-EXUPÉRY

If you're anything like me, choosing Game 2 feels about as attractive as using a cactus for a bath towel. Why would anyone willingly court risk and loss? However, if the Gary Parker Rule has started to convince you that, perhaps, your moving sidewalk isn't taking you where you want to go, you'll eventually have to make that choice.

In the meantime, practice it. Practice risk by trying new things, setting concrete goals, taking small chances, and committing loosely.

IN THE SUMMER OF 2017, Max Deutsch, the co-founder of Monthly.com, decided to master the *New York Times* crossword puzzle.

It wasn't something he'd ever done before. He didn't choose it because he was a natural crossword aficionado. On the contrary: he chose the *New York Times* crossword specifically because he didn't think he could do it.

As he writes, "Crossword puzzles are one of the few things that can't be mastered in any systematic way.... Naturally, I see this as a challenge."[1]

Max's attempt to master the *New York Times* crossword puzzle serves as a spectacular metaphor for preparing ourselves to leave the moving sidewalk. Though it may not always feel like it, our brains love new challenges. In 2014, researchers showed that something as simple as acquiring novel vocabulary words triggered the brain's core reward processing centers. That is, we derive actual, biochemical pleasure from trying something new.

THE *NEW YORK TIMES* crossword puzzle follows a predictable pattern. According to Will Shortz, its editor, anybody can solve a Monday puzzle.[2] Difficulty increases throughout the week, peaking on Saturday. Sunday puzzles are easier, but their grids are bigger.

Max wanted to *master* the puzzle, but what does it mean to master the *New York Times* crossword puzzle? How would Max know if he'd done it? On the other hand, how would he know when to declare failure?

"Try new things," by itself, is problematic advice because it's vague, and vague goals never succeed. How can they?

They sure do tantalize, however. Every New Year's Eve, we fall prey to their wiles. Over half of Americans resolve to save money every year, and 45 percent want to "get fit."[3]

And for obvious reasons: we spend over $1,000, per person, every holiday season.[4] We gain a pound and a half in weight between Halloween and Christmas—which we don't lose again until the following summer.[5] As short-term reactions to holiday remorse, vague New Year's Eve resolutions feel compelling. But what does it mean to "get fit"? What does it mean to "save money"? How do we know when we've succeeded?

More often than not, we don't. Eighty percent of New Year's resolutions fail within six weeks,[6] and I suspect their ambiguity is why. If we haven't set an objective standard against which we can measure our goals, success will always be just out of reach, and we will always feel like perpetual failures. We'll give up.

Max studies learning. He knew this. To stave off ambiguity, he made his goal concrete. He would claim success only if he could finish a Saturday puzzle in one sitting, without any hints or clues, within a month.

This solidifies three things for Max's new challenge: it defines what success means (finishing a Saturday puzzle); it sets constraints (one sitting, no clues); and it delineates a time frame (within a month).

Max's goal was what scientists call *falsifiable*. The only way something can be known to be true—the only way Max could know if he'd mastered the puzzle—is if it *could* be proven false. Either Max would solve a Saturday crossword puzzle in one sitting without clues within a month—or he wouldn't. His hypothesis that he could do it would either be shown to be true, or it wouldn't. It was falsifiable.

A falsifiable hypothesis is far scarier than simply vowing to "get fit" every January, only to chuckle knowingly when we've been to the gym twice by Valentine's Day. It's far scarier than just deciding to change our lives, or to be a better person, or to turn over a new leaf, or even to solve for why.

A falsifiable goal opens the door to failure. We're tempted not to set falsifiable goals but we forget: nonfalsifiable, amorphous goals *guarantee* failure, because success is undefined.

So, try new things, and, in doing so, set falsifiable goals. Whatever the new thing is—mastering the *New York Times* crossword puzzle, becoming a better athlete, spending more time with your children, becoming better at your job—give it concrete parameters.

Make it something you could actually fail. Because if you can fail, then you can succeed.

IN THE SUMMER OF 2017, Alex Honnold became the first person to free-solo Yosemite's El Capitan.* In just under four hours, he climbed three thousand vertical feet of granite without ropes or supports: just him, his shoes, his chalk bag, and his fingers. One mistake would have cost Alex his life.

What he accomplished that day is sweaty-palms amazing. So far, it hasn't been replicated. It's also qualitatively different than what Max accomplished. Alex could have died pursuing his goal; Max, not so much.

But both could have failed.

Decision scientists evaluate choices across two domains:

---

* A little climbing lingo is in order here: rock climbing isn't a single sport. There's trad climbing, sport climbing, top-roping, bouldering, speed climbing—and then there's the insane sport of free-soloing. Most climbing is free-climbing, in that climbers use nothing but their own power to ascend. But most climbers use protection: ropes for big walls or crash pads for boulders. Free-soloers, like Alex Honnold, do away with those. Like all climbers, they ascend under their own power, but, unlike the rest of us, they eschew any safety mechanisms.

the *probability* of any outcome occurring, and the *magnitude* of the outcome if it happens. Though the Gary Parker Rule focuses on the latter, decision theorists claim that humans decide based on both.

Take advantage of this dichotomy.

Free-soloing El Capitan scores poorly on both domains. Although Alex prepared for two years, his probability of falling off the rock remained higher than most of us would accept, and there's no worse outcome than death.

And you know what? Sometimes solving for why will feel exactly like scaling a rock face with no rope. The next two chapters, in fact, are all about failure. So, I'd be lying if I claimed that the road in front of you won't eventually require you to make some El Capitan–sized decisions.

But don't start with them.

When we think about risk, most of us think only about El Capitan, and not about the *New York Times* crossword. We conflate probability with outcome, equating risk with high-likelihood, catastrophic things. And we—wisely—shy away. No one wants to fall off El Capitan.

But Alex didn't start by climbing El Capitan right away. He took small-outcome risks first so that, even if he failed, he'd still be alive.

Max's goal was also quite risky. In fact, he was likely to fail: the Saturday crossword is very hard. The probability side of things wasn't in Max's favor, just like it wasn't in Alex's. Risk faced them both.

On the other hand, the magnitude side was. No matter how much not meeting a goal stings, Max wouldn't have died if he failed.

Do the same. Split the choice dichotomy. Don't think El Capitan; think crosswords. Practice taking risks with floaties on. Practice falling over a net. Pick a task with a substantive *probability* of failure—something you're not sure you can do, something falsifiable—but pick something with nonlethal *outcomes*.

You can't vault off the moving sidewalk if your first jump kills you. So, start risky, but start small.

FINALLY, LEARN TO DANCE. Mikhail Baryshnikov describes ballet as "beautiful, light, and lovely."[7] Crosswords have taught me a lot about trying new things, setting concrete goals, and rethinking risk. They've also taught me to dance. They've taught me to stay light.

Let me give an example. In the *New York Times* crossword puzzle for Saturday, September 15, 2018, David Liben-Nowell clued the five-letter 37-Across with one word: "Skedaddle." A flurry of five-letter options fits this clue. *Leave, split, scoot, scram, go out, speed, hurry.*

When I first started solving crosswords, this openness was paralyzing. What was I supposed to do with all these possibilities? If I chose the wrong one, the puzzle would never be solved, but how could I know what the right choice was?

Fundamentally, however, crosswords allow only two actions: either I could write something down, or I could choose not to. If I didn't, the clue would be wasted, and I'd be no closer to finishing the puzzle. But if I did, there was an 86 percent chance I'd pick the wrong five-letter solution.

This is how I learned to dance.

In 1974, Amos Tversky and Daniel Kahneman published

a paper on the biases that underpin human decision-making.*
They demonstrated one bias, which they called *anchoring*, in an
absolutely brilliant experiment. They gave two groups of high
school students five seconds to estimate the solution to either

$$1 \times 2 \times 3 \times 4 \times 5 \times 6 \times 7 \times 8$$
or
$$8 \times 7 \times 6 \times 5 \times 4 \times 3 \times 2 \times 1$$

Half the students saw the first multiplication problem;
the other half saw the second. The two are mathematically
identical—they both equal 40,320—but Tversky and Kahneman weren't after the right answer. They wanted the students'
first impression, and the difference in those impressions was
enormous.

The group that saw the first string of multiplications guessed
512, on average. The second group guessed 2,250. Neither
group got the right answer—which isn't surprising because they
had only five seconds to respond—but the difference in how
wrong they were caught Tversky and Kahneman's attention.

The researchers hypothesized that the fourfold difference in
the students' estimates emerged because of anchoring. Since we
read from left to right, and since $1 \times 2 \times 3$ is smaller than 8×7
$\times 6$, the first group of students anchored on a smaller number
than the second, and this affected their final guesses.[8]

Anchoring is everywhere. Retailers, for example, use it to
their benefit. In *Priceless: The Myth of Fair Value*, William

---

* Kahneman won a Nobel Prize for this research. Tversky would have but he
had already died when the prize was awarded, and the Nobel committee doesn't
award posthumously.

Poundstone tells the story of a $279 bread maker sold by Williams-Sonoma. No one was buying it—because who in their right mind would spend $279 on a bread maker?

Instead of dropping its price, however, the retailer took advantage of anchoring. It introduced an even more expensive bread maker, stocking the $429 machine right next to the original on their shelves.

No one bought the more expensive bread maker—because who in their right mind would spend over $400 on a bread maker? But sales of the $279 machine doubled. If a $429 model exists, our anchoring bias argues, then $279 feels way cheaper.

Anchoring has obvious connections to crosswords, as well. Any solution to 37-Across—say, *leave*—immediately triggers an anchoring bias. No matter how uncertain I may have felt before I wrote the answer down, the very act of writing *leave* into the grid anchors me, and it affects the rest of the puzzle.

Sharing its first letter with 37-Across is 37-Down. Liben-Nowell clued that six-letter word with "One looking for a hand." Because I've already written *leave* into 37-Across, I'm automatically tempted to find any word that starts with *L* for 37-Down. Unfortunately, none of *lender*, *loaner*, or *loafer* seems appropriate. Instead of rethinking 37-Across, however, anchoring convinces me that, somehow, a *lender* is someone looking for a hand. Before long, I'm five clues in, and the puzzle has ground to a halt.

Because I anchored.

The better way to solve crosswords is to dance. It's to stay light. It's to commit, but to do so loosely. It's to make a decision, but to hold it with an open palm.

The way to dance with crosswords is to write something down—because if not, the grid stays blank and the puzzle never gets solved—but not to anchor. It's to keep other options nearby, so that when it becomes clear that a *suitor* is more likely to be looking for a hand than a *lender,* I'm not stuck.*

Doctors are taught to do this (though, famously, we're not great at it).[9] When a doctor diagnoses a patient with strep throat, she does so with implicit uncertainty. Out loud, she tells the patient, "You have strep throat." To herself, however, she thinks, *You might also have infectious mononucleosis, herpetic stomatitis, aphthous stomatitis, laryngopharyngeal reflux, or, maybe, cancer. Or you could have one of a dozen other diagnoses I haven't even considered.*

She keeps this list of other possibilities nearby. Just as crossword solvers must dance, she must too. She must toe the hairthin line between anchoring—between making a diagnosis and never letting it go—and not committing at all.

She has to diagnose, because what use would she be as a doctor if she didn't? But she must also hold her diagnosis loosely, always considering that she might be wrong. She has to stay light on her metaphorical feet. Any physician who does otherwise, who either never makes a decision or anchors on her initial diagnosis, is bound to make catastrophic mistakes.

THE HAIR-THIN LINE BETWEEN committing too strongly and not committing at all is ubiquitous. In 2013, Reshma Saujani ran for a congressional seat to represent New York State. She didn't win,† but in her travels across the state she incidentally noticed a gender gap in computing classes. Boys took them; girls didn't.

---

* The correct answer to 37-Across, by the way, was *split*; 37-Down was *suitor.*
† Reshma calls this failed run transformative. It pushed her off her own moving sidewalk and toward her why.

In response, she founded Girls Who Code, aimed at providing programming experience to middle and high school girls.[10] It's been enormously successful: over 90 percent of its participants want to major in computer science, compared to the 4 percent of female college freshmen who do.

Saujani observed that programming teeters on the same hair-thin line. Coding can be frustratingly nitpicky. Entire programs are at the mercy of a single misplaced semicolon. Saujani saw two responses to this finickiness. When some students—girls more often than boys—asked her for help, they showed her a blank screen, as if they'd never tried anything. She learned to click Undo on these blank screens, because when she did, hours of work appeared. Unwilling to commit, the student had decided to delete her work before showing the teacher. She preferred a blank screen to a mistake. These students wouldn't even step out on the dance floor.

Other students fell on the opposite side of the line. They anchored. When the computer didn't perform the way they wanted, these kids choked. I've seen this mistake a lot among some of my own research assistants, as well. Research involves a good bit of coding, and I've had mentees write frustrated, desperately anchored emails: "I *know* this code is right, but I can't figure out why it doesn't work."

Despite incontrovertible evidence to the contrary—computers only do what they're told—these students and researchers are convinced their code is correct. They've committed, but they've done it too tightly. Unlike the students with blank screens, these coders are at least on the dance floor. But they aren't light.

Coding, crossword puzzles, and medicine require dancing on the hair-thin line between anchoring and not choosing, because either committing too tightly or not committing at all can create stagnation.

As Doe Zantamata writes, "We can think about things, turn them over in our minds a million times, play out possible scenarios, but really when it comes down to it, you have to go with your heart and move forward. Maybe things will go well. Maybe they'll turn out poorly.... The only thing that's for sure is that indecision steals many years from many people who wind up wishing they'd just had the courage to leap."[11]

Chapter 16

Don't judge me by my successes. Judge me by how
many times I fell down and got back up again.

—NELSON MANDELA

IN 2015, EIGHT PEOPLE gathered around the diminutive, five-year-old body of a girl dwarfed by her hospital bed. Lines ran from her arms and legs to whirring pumps that pushed the drugs keeping her heart beating, her blood pressure stable, and any infections at bay. A tube traced its serpentine course from her trachea to the larger, louder machine that forced pure oxygen into her lungs.

But Benedictine had already gone.

Her pupils refused to respond to my penlight. She didn't flinch at painful stimuli. Her kidneys had stopped working the day before, and she'd lost her respiratory drive. I'd already discussed next steps with her mother. She didn't want to be in the room when it happened.

The charge nurse disconnected the ventilator, turned off its insistent, sustained alarm. The room descended into a dense, woolly silence.

For an uncomfortably long time, Benedictine's vital signs remained normal. Then, her blood oxygen level floated downward and, with it, her heart rate. Minutes passed. The numbers settled to zero.

An embracing stillness greeted the stethoscope I laid on her chest. The comforting double pulse of a beating heart and the papery waves of air moving through alveoli were glaringly absent. At five forty in the evening, on a warm March day in a port city in sub-Saharan Africa, the darkness won.

BENEDICTINE HAD BEEN BORN with a vascular malformation. A disordered growth of veins in her face formed a lake of blood over her right jaw. They infiltrated the bone itself, swelling her jaw to the size of an avocado.

She'd had three prior surgeries, each meant to sclerose the malformation—to replace it with enough scar tissue that we could access, and remodel, the deformed mandibular bone beneath it.

Three prior times, she had visited the windowless room on the third deck of the hospital ship. Three prior times, she'd been put to sleep. Three prior times, a surgeon submersed the pinpoint tip of an electrocautery pencil into her tumor, tuning its current precisely to replace the malformed vessels with scar. Three prior times, she'd woken up. Three prior times, she'd been wheeled back to the recovery room, wrapped in a viridian blanket. Three prior times, she'd been returned to her mother.

Her fourth trip should have been no different.

The Dutch operating room nurse fetched Benedictine from the wards. Together with a ward nurse, a translator, and Benedictine's mother, they prayed for safety on the operating table.

My plan that day was simple: elevate skin, soft tissue, and

scar, and recontour the underlying bone. It's as straightforward a procedure as we do on that hospital ship. Because the jaw swelling was benign, I didn't have to take it all out. All I had to do was to restore symmetry to Benedictine's face.

The nursing team wheeled her across the fire doors separating the wards from the surgical suite. After we confirmed her name, birth date, hospital ID, and the name and location of the procedure, the anesthesiologist put Benedictine to sleep.

We moved with the ease of a team that had been working together for years, because many of us had. We prepped her with a russet antiseptic solution and unfolded blue drapes over her tiny body. Her humanity obscured, Benedictine and her tumor became a task I had done hundreds of times before and have done hundreds of times since. Knife entered skin, muscles unfurled upward, and, within minutes, the deformed jaw emerged, ivory, mottled, and riddled with holes, as if moths had eaten it.

The nurse readied the drill, tested it, primed the water, and prepared the suction. Under its scalloped burr, bone melted, and from the overgrowth a new jaw began to take shape.

"Mark, could you stop for a second?" The soft, British-accented voice of the anesthesiologist.

Without warning, Benedictine's blood pressure had plummeted. In seconds, we rewound our prep. We tore the drapes, covered her surgical wound, and rolled the crash cart into the room.

Her pulse had disappeared. I started chest compressions. Anesthesiologists, nurses, and surgeons from other operating rooms poured in. The chief anesthesiologist began calling out instructions from the pediatric advanced life support protocol.

As Benedictine's body shook under the compressions, other

doctors pumped it full of a pharmacopeia of cardiac drugs. Everyone's focus narrowed to their single task. Mine was simply to push blood around her body because her heart wouldn't. "Come on," I muttered. "Come on. Come on. Come on."

As her pulse returned, her spirit whispered its farewell. The protocol worked, but she was gone.

Benedictine officially didn't die on the operating table. She died in the ICU three days later. The ship's carpenters fashioned her a coffin. A missionary family donated a new dress for her burial. Another charity offered a helicopter to fly her and her mother back to their village in the north.

A tangle of emotions surrounds a patient's death; chief among them is shame. For days, I couldn't meet anyone's eye. I felt like those eyes accused me of killing a five-year-old girl. I accused me too.

Sure, we held our regular morbidity and mortality conference later that week. Sure, we concluded that, with the tools available to us on that hospital ship, we did everything we could. Sure, we could never definitively determine why her blood pressure dropped. We couldn't do an autopsy, and nothing in her five-year-old history predicted any risk.

Sure.

But one fact resisted rational analysis: had I not taken Benedictine to the operating room, she would still be alive. She was alive until I messed with her. Alive until I tried to fix things.

ALMOST A DECADE BEFORE Benedictine died, I had solved for why. Four years before, I left the moving sidewalk. I knew I was where I wanted to be, living a life my younger self would have been proud of.

And in the middle of it, a five-year-old lost her life.

Was Benedictine's death truly my fault? James Reason would argue that it wasn't. In 2000, Reason proposed a Swiss cheese model for medical errors.[1]

Before Reason, medicine viewed errors as a single person's fault. An adverse outcome for a patient had to be attributed to a responsible party—the surgeon whose knife slipped, the nurse who misdosed a patient, the pharmacist who didn't catch it. "Naturally enough," Reason wrote, "associated countermeasures are directed mainly at reducing unwanted variability in human behavior," through the creation of process maps, the legislation of algorithms, or the threat of lawsuits.

Reason suggested that, instead, medical errors were failures of a system, not a person. "Although some unsafe acts in any sphere are egregious," he wrote, "the vast majority are not. In aviation maintenance . . . some 90 percent of quality lapses were judged as blameless." If 90 percent of errors are blameless, he reasoned, then looking for a scapegoat wouldn't make patients any safer.

In the Swiss cheese model, not every slipped knife or incorrect dosage leads to adverse outcomes, because the system protects its patients. Machines alarm. Beds have railings. Dangerous medications have to be countersigned by two people. Electronic medical records flag allergies.

And most of the time, these defenses work. "However," he wrote, the defenses "are more like slices of Swiss cheese, having many holes—though unlike in the cheese, these holes are continually opening, shutting, and shifting their location."

Adverse outcomes—even those that leave a five-year-old comatose in the ICU—occur because ephemeral Swiss cheese holes line up for an inauspicious nanosecond. The alarm fails to beep at the same time that the nurse happens to look away and the doctor is with a different patient.

It took a while for Reason's model to stick, but he's right. Most medical errors aren't the result of egregious malfeasance by a single person. When I was a medical student, morbidity and mortality conferences felt like a medieval inquisition. Students presented the week's mortalities to a panel of wise surgeons arrayed in the front row of a dark auditorium. Every week, their leader, a loud, Napoleonic character, warranted that, if only he'd done the case, the patient would still be alive. Wasn't it such a shame, the residents' silent assent declared, that the medical student had been so clumsy?

Now, instead of kowtowing to short, strident surgeons, we talk about Swiss cheese. We diagnose system breakdowns. We discuss physical infrastructure, organizational ethos, communication, and supply chains. It's definitely made patients safer.

And it's also allowed us to abdicate responsibility for failure.

Properly Swiss-cheesed, failure becomes edentulous. If an unfortunate alignment of constantly shifting holes led to Benedictine's death, then no one could be held individually accountable. She died because the system let her down.

Swiss cheese distances us from our outcomes, and we're grateful for it.

UNLESS, OF COURSE, THOSE outcomes are good. Then they're ours. We'd rather ascribe success to ourselves and failure to Swiss cheese.

In 2016, a colleague removed a massive, congenital neck tumor from a Beninese man named Innocent. Innocent recovered slowly; his wound required daily dressing changes. Thanks to meticulous nursing care, he improved for twenty-two days. On the morning of the twenty-third day, he complained of transient neck pain, which disappeared by the afternoon.

By the evening, blood saturated his nurse, his neighbor, and the ceiling above them. Innocent lost liters in minutes; it covered the walls, the sheets, and his caretaker. A brewing neck infection had eroded into an artery, and, that night, it exploded.

Dr. Lindsay Sherriff, a former general practitioner from the Australian outback, was on call. He flattened Innocent into his bed, lifted the patient's ankles onto his own shoulders, and jammed his fist into the bleeding man's belly.

This move tamponaded Innocent's aorta, forcing blood upward toward his brain. It's a risky maneuver: Innocent could have lost his legs or his kidneys to hypoxia, but Dr. Sherriff reasoned that life with an amputation was better than death.

And he saved Innocent's life.

As did the system. While the blood-soaked nurse held pressure on the patient's neck and Dr. Sherriff held pressure on his belly, the operating room team readied the emergency OR. The ward team wheeled his gurney into the waiting theater. The blood bank lined up donors. Chaplains found Innocent's family. The first surgeon to respond took over from the nurse, holding pressure until reinforcements arrived.

We knew that night that once pressure was removed from Innocent's neck, we may never regain control. We might be powerless to keep him from dying.

Vascular blowouts like Innocent's carry a 10 percent risk of stroke.[2] In my career, I've seen two patients die of them.

Innocent, however, walked out of the hospital, thanks both to Dr. Sherriff's fist in his belly and to a system that worked.

EVERY FAILURE IS THE result of a complex interplay of individual choices and the systems in which they're made. So, too, is every success.

Because of how ubiquitous they are, however, systems are easy to blame. By ascribing responsibility for our failures to them, we create what psychologists have called an external locus of control. Instead of embracing failure for what it is, we take cover under this external locus, shifting blame to an anonymous outside, while assigning to ourselves the credit for any success.

We carry this external locus into our career decisions as well. It's easy, for example, to blame the moving sidewalk for choices that have kept us on it, because we make these choices while on the very same sidewalk.

It doesn't help that solving for why is no protection against catastrophe. Worse: it actually forces us to confront the exact things the external locus of control is specifically designed to avoid—failure, anxiety, and doubt. I keep insinuating that, off the moving sidewalk, we also find wonder, faith, and worship, but we've got to face those three demons first before we can get there.

Brené Brown writes, "Daring is not saying 'I'm willing to risk failure.' Daring is saying 'I know I will eventually fail, and I'm still all in.'"[3]

That's heavy stuff: I *know* I will eventually fail.

Failure is guaranteed off the moving sidewalk. It doesn't have be as lethal or as public as mine for it to mess with our heads. No matter how small it is, we still do all we can to avoid it. That's what makes the moving sidewalk so attractive in the first place. I stayed on it for as long as I did, even though I hated it, because I wasn't all in.

You, too, may hate your moving sidewalk. It may fill you with gut-numbing angst. You may want to be anywhere but in your day-to-day. But you're on that sidewalk because you're at least decent at it. You've gotten good at living your personal monotony. As much as the moving sidewalk may be responsible for feelings of loss or for inchoate dissatisfaction, you wouldn't be stuck on it if you couldn't accomplish its demands.

But Dr. Brown is right: once you leave it, you're going to fail. It's a guarantee. You *will* find yourself flat on your face at some point. It may not be in an operating room on a hospital ship, and it may not cost a five-year-old her life, but I guarantee it's going to hurt.

You could recoil from it and stay safe under the protection of an external locus of control. You could blame anyone but yourself for it. But if failure happens *to* you—while you create your success—then you'll never solve for why.

Chapter 17

It's impossible to live without failing at something, unless you live so cautiously that you might as well not have lived at all—in which case you fail by default.

—J. K. ROWLING

O NE NIGHT, IN A fit of hubris, I auditioned for *American Ninja Warrior*, a television show that pits athletes against an obstacle course. Like many doctors, I grew up introverted, bookish, and unathletic. An ideal weekend for preteen me involved maneuvering a pixelated knight through dragon-slaying, treasure-hunting conquests.

I got into one and only one playground fight in grade school. It ended with me suffocating under the substantial body of my opponent, his punches reminding me that nerds always lose.

My parents, God bless them, tried to turn me into a semi-competent athlete. They put me in tennis lessons, but I could never overcome the ball's magnetic attraction to the net. They tried swim lessons, and I chose to swim breaststroke because it was the easiest.

They put me on the soccer team, where I opted to play defense, because defenders ran the least. In high school, my entire class tried out for the football team. Everyone got a position (probably because our homeroom teacher was also the football coach). Some of my friends were on the defensive line. One of them became the quarterback.

I was the water boy.

To put it simply, I wasn't an athlete. Also, I really loved cheese, donuts, Wendy's burgers, Mounds bars, and Oreos. By the time I was thirty-five, I was overweight. I reasoned that fact away: single indicators like weight don't, for example, consider muscle mass (not that I had much of that either). And even if heart disease and cancer run in my family—both of which are unequivocally associated with excess fat—I felt healthy enough.

At thirty-five, I discovered rock climbing, and I took to it like I take to donuts. It's the perfect introvert sport. Some days could just be me against the wall. Others, I'd spend socializing with any of the dozen climbers trying to master the chess of moving our bodies across an overhang.

Gradually, my love for the sport transformed my relationship with my body. As I became more confident in my climbing, I became more serious about my health. Stronger at forty-one than I was at twenty-five, I made a rash, two-o'clock-in-the-morning decision to apply for *American Ninja Warrior*. After six years of climbing, I figured an obstacle course couldn't be that hard.

Eight pages of probing questions and a three-minute video later, I submitted my application. Casting receives seventy-five thousand applications a year, so I forgot about mine. There was no way they'd pick a forty-one-year-old, bookish surgeon from Boston.

You don't get a lot of warning with *American Ninja Warrior*. I got an unofficial call from the producers six weeks before filming—the official call to compete would come three weeks later—and I hadn't yet been on a single ninja obstacle.

Still, I did well enough on the show that year, and an obsession was born. I love the sport because I love the things it forces me to do. I love watching this aging body prove that anyone—even the kid who was barely fit enough to be the water boy—can be an athlete.

And, I love that it's forced me to fail. A lot.

THREE YEARS AFTER I first set foot on the *American Ninja Warrior* course, I was scheduled to tackle it a third time. Not many people get three opportunities, especially if, like me, their performances don't improve each year.

In 2016, I had little to prove. I'd only been training for a few weeks, so no matter how far I got on the course, it would have been a victory. My run wasn't aired, but I didn't mind because I knew I'd come back, better trained, and better prepared to complete the course the next year.

That first year, pre-competition jitters inexplicably disappeared right before I ran. I walked to the starting block focused, tranquil, and ready. The next year, in 2017, I expected the same flow state.

Three runners before I was scheduled to go, my heart still raced. Two runners, and my legs felt leaden. Then, without warning, the competitor before me fell early, and it was my turn. I walked to the starting block tense, nervous, and slow. I told myself I was anxious because the course is hard. Truth is, however, I was nervous because I needed to prove to the producers that I'd improved. I had to beat my first performance.

I didn't. I did worse. That night, I cried over a year of training that culminated in twenty seconds on the course.

The producers didn't call me to compete in 2018. I know of four surgeons, including myself, who compete in ninja events. The other three got the call that year, which told me all I needed to know: I'd blown my chances.

Fair enough too. I wouldn't have given myself a third chance, and I wouldn't expect the producers to either. More than a sport, *American Ninja Warrior* is a TV show. Producers want good stories and athletes they can invest in—and I hadn't proved to be a solid investment.

When I applied in 2019, it was a throwaway application. Inexplicably, the producers disagreed.

"Congratulations!" one of them said when he called. "You've been selected to compete on *American Ninja Warrior* season 11!" He'd say this to six hundred other competitors that month. He was tired. I'm convinced I would have made his job easier had I turned his offer down.

But Grandpa Finlay wouldn't have turned him down. So, I hid my fear from the producer and said yes. I hid it from my family, from my friends, and, most especially, from my public persona. "So excited," my social media posts said. "I can't wait to test my mettle against that course for the third time."

That was a lie. I'd struggled that year with a deep-set inadequacy. In the middle of writing *Solving for Why*, I wrestled with reservations about my own bona fides.

In local and regional ninja competitions, it's not uncommon

for athletes to fall on early obstacles. It happens to everyone, but it happened a lot more frequently to me because I'd psych myself out. *If you fall early*, the voices in my head would argue, *you won't have to face the scarier, later obstacles. And you can finally stop pretending you're actually an athlete. What a ridiculous idea, anyway, this athlete thing! You do nerdy things. You play computer games. You write research papers. People like you aren't athletes. You learned that lesson on the playground.*

At the same time, I knew the producer's invitation meant I'd be back on the starting block two years after the course defeated me. So, I threw myself into preparation. I devoured sports psychology books. I lived at the gym. I ripped the skin on my hands, taped them up, and ripped again through the tape. By the time I faced the obstacle course on May 24, 2019, in Cincinnati, I was stronger than I'd ever been.

As a sport, ninja warrior can be distilled into a small movement repertoire. Obstacles differ, but success relies on a few skills: Can you stay light on your feet? Can you do a bunch of pull-ups? Can you kip your hips high enough to create a split second of weightlessness? Can you throw your body across a gap in front of you? Can you do it sideways?

Like all ninjas, I'm better at some movements than others, and I got lucky in Cincinnati. The course they had designed required only the skills I was good at. Six obstacles lay between me and the final buzzer, and I knew I could complete them all.

I was ready.

American Ninja Warrior films overnight. Ninety-seven competitors ran before I hit the starting block at four thirty in the morning on May 25. Many of them had finished the course.

I was ready to join them.

With ten runners to go, the line producer took me to the warm-up area. I went through my routine. Lateral hops. Pull-ups. Push-ups. Core activation.

I was ready.

Five runners to go, and I felt limber. My pulse was in the right place. My joints were lubricated, my muscles warm.

I was ready.

I walked up the steps to the starting block.

I was ready.

I waved to my family on the sidelines and felt the rush of adrenaline.

And then I wasn't ready.

I wanted to run, but I was trapped. There was a show to film, a course to tackle, obstacles to complete. And I wasn't ready.

The line producer counted me down, and I wasn't ready. I saw five shrinking steps and the rope I'd have to grab to complete the first obstacle, and I wasn't ready. The producer told me to go.

And I wasn't ready.

Three steps into the first obstacle, I failed. I froze, and, like a wide-eyed cat, I retreated. I didn't fall off the course so much as simply step off it.

Two years of preparation, two years to improve, and my performance could no longer be measured by *which* obstacle defeated me, but by how many steps I took before chickening out.

Not a single competitor did worse than I did that night. Cincinnati validated what I suspected: I was a fraud.

The crowd knew it. The producers knew it. My fellow competitors knew it. For three years, ninja training had been about being more than a water boy.

And I failed.

I STRUGGLED TO EXPLAIN away Cincinnati like I wanted to Swiss-cheese Benedictine's death: it was after four o'clock in the morning, I was tired, I was cold, I had a panic attack. Not one of these is wrong, but each prevents me from doing what I need to do with failure.

I need to fall in love with it.

Not just to accept it or to endure it, but to fall in actual love with failing.

Let me be the first to admit: failure sucks. It deeply, viscerally sucks. It would be easy to write glibly about how important failure is for growth, easy to encourage myself just to buck up, to keep my chin up, to stiffen my upper lip, to stay positive. It would be easy for any discussion on failure to devolve into platitudinous positivity without paying homage to the fact that failure is, by definition, failure. It is soul crushing.

IT'S ALSO THE COST of admission. "I've never met a brave person," Brené Brown writes, "who hasn't known disappointment, failure, even heartbreak."[1]

You, too, will fail if you leave the moving sidewalk. And that is a beautiful thing.

I've learned to fall in love with failure not because failure is pleasant, but because it is beautiful. Failure tells me I tried something I don't yet know how to do. It indicates I'm moving. And it shows me that I'm no longer on the anodyne path.

How thrilling is that?

Failure will still punch you in the gut. It'll still suck. But you have two choices: you can avoid it—which you can only accomplish by staying on the moving sidewalk—or you can change your stance toward it. Instead of seeing it as a challenge, instead of making it something to endure or to overcome, instead of gritting your teeth and hoping you fail as little as possible, you can, instead, fall in love with failure's beauty.

THREE DECADES AGO, CAROL Dweck, a psychologist at Stanford University, asked ten-year-olds to solve math problems slightly above their ability.[2] In other words, she purposely made them fail.

They responded in two ways. One group found their inevitable failure soul destroying. The very existence of these math problems proved what the students always suspected about themselves. It wasn't just that they couldn't *do* the problems. It was that they *were* the sort of students who couldn't do the problems. That these problems even existed meant that there were people who could solve them—people who were, fundamentally, better. The problems threatened who the students were, not just what they could accomplish.

Dr. Dweck's problems inspired the second group. To them, the problems didn't represent existential catastrophe. They represented *not yet*, a level they would one day attain, even if, today, they failed. They agreed with the first group: if these problems existed, there were people out there who could solve them. But they went one step further. They added hope. If people existed who could solve the problems, these students could join them one day.

The first group couldn't solve Dweck's problems. The second group couldn't solve Dweck's problems—*yet*. To the first group, failure meant that they were fundamentally flawed. To the second, the problems were evidence of a world they had yet to unlock.

Dweck theorized—and further research has supported—that future success depended on which mindset the students adopted: the *fixed mindset* of the first group or the *growth mindset* of the second.

Failure for growth mindsets represents possibility; failure for fixed mindsets represents personal judgment. Our mindsets dictate our responses to challenges and to uncertainty. Where fixed mindsets see opportunities to prove how terrible they are, growth mindsets see opportunities to improve. Where fixed mindsets can immediately list all the ways they'll mess up a challenge, growth mindsets see hope. They see *yet*.

Three things characterize growth mindsets.

First, they predispose the people who have them to believing in malleability. Nothing is fixed, not social attributes, not personality, not intelligence, ability, faith—or even the mindset itself.

Second, although growth mindsets lead to better results, people with growth mindsets aren't results-oriented. That's counterintuitive; we're initiated into the worship of results from childhood. And for good reason: we want our surgeons and our airline pilots to be results-oriented. "I tried my best" isn't enough to land a 737.

It's more than enough for ourselves, however. We aren't 737s. A lot is out of our control, especially once we step off the moving sidewalk. Progress can be frustratingly nonlinear, so focusing only on *getting* to where we think we should go becomes paralyzing.

For people with growth mindsets, remaining results-independent instead of results-oriented girds them against inevitable failures. Thomas Merton, an American Trappist monk and Zen practitioner, once wrote, "Do not depend on the hope of results.... You may have to face the fact that your work will be apparently worthless and even achieve...results opposite to what you expect. As you get used to this idea you start more and more to concentrate not on the results but on the value, the rightness, the truth of the work itself."[3]

"Do not depend on the hope of results"—which is precisely what we're all raised to depend on! We genuflect before the hope of results. It's part of the ethos of Work. Merton cautions against this idolatry: focus instead, he says, on value, on rightness, and on truth. Focus on the why, even if the why gives you results that go against everything you'd hoped to accomplish.

Finally, because they're not results-oriented and because they believe everything is malleable, people with growth mindsets adopt a learner's posture. Instead of consequence, they pursue competence.

As a result, they actively seek challenge, and even woo failure, viewing obstacles as an opportunity to test their mettle and to get better. They understand that only by putting themselves in the path of failure can they become what they want to be. And in doing so, sometimes they fall in love with failure itself—because failure is the incarnation of *yet*.

On the other hand, people with fixed mindsets pursue performance. They want to get it right, and challenges are an opportunity to get it very, very wrong. Because they pursue perfection, people with fixed mindsets cower from negative feedback. Every challenge becomes an occasion for the world to find them lacking, every barrier a test of their worth, every obstacle a chance for them to prove what they already know: they're impostors.

Far safer to stay on the moving sidewalk, because there, they can't fail. There, they're perfect. "The idea of perfection all too often sabotages our ability to become who we have the potential to be," writes Ryder Carroll. "We're marvelous yet imperfect creatures."[4]

If these three characteristics—a belief in malleability, results independence, and a learner's posture—distinguish people with a growth mindset from their more fixed counterparts, one characteristic does not: innate ability.

Dweck's research has shown unequivocally that initial ability does not correlate with mindset. It's not the case that the smartest students have growth mindsets or that failure breeds a fixed mindset. "Indeed," she writes in a paper she co-authored with Ellen Leggett at Harvard, "some of the brightest, most skilled individuals exhibit the maladaptive pattern."[5]

In other words, failure doesn't lead to a fear of failure, and a fear of failure doesn't lead to success. Just the opposite. Our attitudes toward failure predate—and eventually shape—our failures.

DURING MY TIME AS a trainee in Toronto, I spent nine months studying under Ralph Gilbert, one of Canada's best microvascular surgeons. To his trainees, Ralph can sometimes feel demanding—but he's exactly the surgeon I'd want to treat me.

The man's a magician. His surgeries are beautiful to watch,

microscopic fugues set to the pulse oximeter's insistent rhythm. He's also lightning-fast. What takes a surgeon like me an hour, he'll do in nineteen minutes.

Ralph's skill is incredible because he's never satisfied. I've seen him ponder minuscule hand movements, debating whether they'll shave a few seconds off his time. He's so good because he's learned from even the smallest misstep. Ralph fails beautifully. He fails correctly. He fails forward.

Bill Hybels, the founding pastor of an American megachurch, calls this attitude *incessant tinkering*.[6] No sermon he preaches is perfect; some are frankly duds. But instead of labeling the duds as failures, Bill keeps tinkering, keeps improving. He, too, fails forward.

Every operation, every sale, every sermon, every written word, every patient, every litigated case, and every tentative decision on the road to why can be either an opportunity for soul-crushing failure, or an opportunity for incessant tinkering. The next operation, sale, word, sermon, patient, or life decision is around the corner.

I LOVE ANIMATED MOVIES, and *Kung Fu Panda* is one of the best. Its protagonist is Po, an idle, clumsy, noodle-selling panda from the Valley of Peace. Although Po daydreams of becoming a kung fu master, he's more pasta than prowess.

When his village is attacked by a snow leopard, however, he's mistakenly chosen to become the next Dragon Warrior. The village sends him to train with his five kung fu idols, their master, Shifu, and Shifu's master, the turtle Oogway.

After a particularly demoralizing training day, Oogway and

Po meet at a peach tree. Oogway asks the neophyte panda why he's so upset.

"I probably sucked more today than anyone in the history of kung fu, in the history of China, in the history of sucking," Po responds.

"Probably," Oogway agrees.

"And the five! Man, you should have seen them. They totally hate me."

"Totally."

"How is Shifu ever going to turn me into the Dragon Warrior? I mean, I'm not like the five. I've got no claws, no wings, no venom…Maybe I should just quit and go back to making noodles."

"Quit. Don't quit. Noodles. Don't noodles. You are too concerned with what was and what will be."

Po's panda mindset is fixed. He wants perfection. When he doesn't see results, he concludes that he sucks, that everyone knows it, that everyone hates him, and that really all he's fit to do is make noodles.

And Oogway agrees! The panda *has* sucked more than anyone in the history of sucking. His five kung fu idols totally *do* hate him.

Oogway's response to Po's fixed mindset is brilliant. He doesn't deny the failure, doesn't pretend Po didn't fail. He owns it, and, by doing so, he tells Po that failure—the very real, very tangible, very sucky failure—is just today. "You are too concerned with what was and what will be," Oogway says. Too concerned, as Merton would have put it, with the hope of results. Too concerned with the outcomes.

To Po, failure means he is inherently incapable of his

dreams. Oogway's reality is different: Po failed—today. He's not like his five idols. Yet.

I HAVE A NATURALLY fixed mindset. Unfortunately, my peach-tree moment didn't involve a wise turtle. It involved a throwaway interaction with a friend.

Derek, a fellow ninja athlete, and I had been training at a local ninja gym one Tuesday night. We ended the session by training balance and agility. I don't like balance obstacles. They're dodgy. They're designed specifically to trip you up. They're also my weakness.

After we set up a particularly tricky balance line, we both looked at each other, and said, "Well, this is a stupid idea." Someone would roll an ankle that night—and for me, that was sufficient. It was dumb. I wanted to work on things I already knew how to do, because they were safer.

It wasn't sufficient for Derek. His sentence didn't end there. "This is a stupid idea," he agreed. And then, mischievously, "I'm in."

And there it was. My fixed mindset *knew* I couldn't do the line we had set up. The obstacles were above my abilities. I was going to fail. Derek would see it. Everyone at the gym would see it. I was about to prove to them all just how bad a failed ninja I was.

Derek, instead, saw the crazy line of obstacles as an opportunity. He could have rolled his ankle that night too—the obstacles were as far outside his skill set as they were outside of mine. He knew he was taking a risk. And he was all in.*

---

* For the record, no ankles were rolled, but we fell. A lot.

The only surgeon without complications is the surgeon who doesn't operate. The arrow hits the gold only after a thousand bounces. Michael Jordan is reported to have said, "I've missed more than 9,000 shots in my career. I've lost almost 300 games. Twenty-six times, I've been trusted to take the game winning shot and missed. I've failed over and over and over again in my life. And that is why I succeed."[7]

The first part of this book documented a decade and a half of what, in the moment, felt like consequential failures: medical school, Singapore, residency, my first clinical job. Each failure should have been the end of my story. I hated those years. I wanted to tell Oogway, "Maybe I should just quit and go back to making noodles." But where I am now is a direct result of those failures. And where you go next will be built on yours.

As bumpy, curvy, and torturous as the path ahead of you looks, "do not," as Thich Nhat Hanh writes, "judge yourself harshly as a failure. Just start again."[8] Will you go back to making noodles, or will you make the scary, intentional decisions you need to move forward? Will you demand perfection, or will you fall in love with failure?

More than your ankle is at risk, you marvelous, imperfect creature.

Are you in?

Chapter 18

Fear walked where it would, and there was no use pretending it away.

—EVAN JAMES

ON SEPTEMBER 14, 2001, I boarded a plane. I'd spend the next fifteen years wrestling with the man who disembarked 210 minutes later.

Moving to New York City for residency three months prior hadn't been my first choice, but doctors don't get to choose their residency programs. Instead, an optimization algorithm matches us to residency slots within our chosen specialty. It's a process as simple as it is opaque.

A graduating medical student applies to as many residencies as she's interested in. Programs interested in her invite her for an in-person interview. After the interview, both the program and the resident create rank lists. The applicant ranks the programs she's visited, in order of how happy she thinks they'd make her, and programs rank the students they invited to interview. Both lists are then fed into a nationwide optimization algorithm, and whatever pairings the computer returns become legally binding.

Ideally, the applicant's rank list should reflect her personal priorities, and programs should consider only the applicants they want to train. Reality is, however, knottier. Doctors are a competitive breed, and the match algorithm jeopardizes our chances to win. Medical schools count it a victory if their graduates match high on their rank lists. Applicants, too, can brag if they match at the places they ranked highly. Residencies win when they accept only their top choices.

Incentives therefore misalign: applicants rank programs based not on how much they like them, but on how likely they are to get in. Residency programs first consider how highly an applicant will rank them before ceding to her a top slot. It's residency Tinder, with less catfishing.

"Every system," wrote W. Edwards Deming, "is perfectly designed to get the results it gets."* This one too. Three-quarters of applicants match within their top three choices.[1] Whether this means that 75 percent of applicants match at programs they best fit, however, is less clear.

Like everyone, I played the residency matching game. I optimized my chances of matching high on my list, instead of ranking programs in the order that I would have liked. Unlike most, however, I didn't succeed.

As a medical student in Texas, New York City was the last

---

* The attribution to Deming is disputed. The original may have come from Drs. Donald Berwick or Paul Batalden. The latter claims credit for this quote, writing that he altered an earlier quote from Arthur Jones: "All organizations are perfectly designed to get the results they get." See Earl Conway and Paul Batalden, "Like Magic? ('Every System Is Perfectly Designed...')," Institute for Healthcare Improvement. August 21, 2015, http://www.ihi.org/communities/blogs/origin-of-every-system-is-perfectly-designed-quote.

place I'd ever wanted to move. I ranked only a few programs lower than Columbia, but that's where the algorithm sent me. So, in June of 2001, I moved to the warm, wet torpor that is summer in the city.

My first apartment was an eighty-one-square-foot room with a single window framing a perpetually belching smoke-stack. The room barely fit a twin bed and a closet; a chipped, oxidized sink cantilevered from the left wall. The entry door just cleared the sink before getting jammed against the bed.

New York may not have been where I wanted to live, but the city gets under your skin. Six months in, either you can't wait to leave, or you can't imagine living anywhere else. I couldn't imagine living anywhere else.

I could walk out of my tiny room at one o'clock in the morn-ing for sushi halfway up the block, at a three-table restaurant run by a man who moved his family from Japan to pursue his shad roe dreams. I could disappear into the peaceful anonym-ity of eight million people.

I could stumble on small house parties, join drum circles in Prospect Park, and befriend the nomadic ninety-year-old lady and her surly puppy who walked my block every morning. I joined a tribe of haggard interns plying the embattled halls of a hospital, priding ourselves on threading intravenous lines through heroin-scarred veins while subsisting on peanut butter and Diet Coke.

New York is an incredible place.

EIGHT FORTY-SIX A.M. ON Tuesday, September 11, 2001, has been chiseled into the national psyche. For eight million New Yorkers, the attacks on the World Trade Center that clear, blue morning were more than a national tragedy. They were an attack on our home. They laid our corner of the universe bare.

For weeks, we could see the smoke from Ground Zero anywhere in the city. One in five Americans knew someone hurt or killed in the September 11 attacks.[2] In New York City, however, that number was much higher.

We united in very public ways—we volunteered at Ground Zero; we gave blood; we took care of victims; we comforted friends; we mourned the lost. But underneath the unity, we were divided by a more private fear. The attacks toppled hardened New Yorkers into anxiety and a terrifying recognition of our vulnerability.

We wouldn't exhale for two years.

The summer of 2003 had been torrid, so when alarm software at an Ohio energy company glitched on August 14, it leveled the electrical grid from Ohio to Ontario, from Michigan to Boston to New York City. All told, darkness covered fifty-five million people that day.

At the ENT clinic at Columbia Presbyterian Hospital, near the northern tip of Manhattan, the power died as we saw our final patients of the afternoon. We carried wheelchair-bound patients down seven flights, made call coverage arrangements, and then joined gridlocked traffic.

In the three hours it took to cover the eight miles between work and home, the sun set. Our apartments, however, broiled. Elevators didn't work. Water pumps failed. We couldn't drink, shower, or flush a toilet. The blackout of 2003 gave us two choices: we could opt to stay home, hoping for an electrical resurrection before we had to pee, or we could hit the streets.

Manhattan hit the streets that night. Music poured from

battery-powered stereos. Bodegas that couldn't keep their ice cream frozen gave it away. We wandered a blacked-out island, in the churn of a million others. We'd never seen stars in New York City before.

It didn't matter who you were on August 14, 2003—just like it didn't matter who you were two years earlier when planes attacked us. That night, you were a New Yorker. That night, you danced in the streets with other New Yorkers, drenched in sweat, hands tacky from melted ice cream, the Milky Way unfurled above, and the sounds of reggaeton in your ears.

The blackout may have cost $6.4 billion,[3] but it gave us our city back.

I'M GETTING AHEAD OF myself.

Most airlines resumed a limited flying schedule on September 13, 2001.[4] I boarded a plane the next day, three days after the World Trade Center attacks. As the pilot maneuvered our half-full plane around the southern end of Manhattan, he tipped the wings, in case anyone wanted to see Ground Zero from above.

I looked. Pillars of ash and smoke still rose from the caldera.

And the panic attack started. As smoke billowed upward, my chest sunk. Tinnitus eclipsed the engine's roar. Seated and seat-belted, I felt like I was falling. My vision tightened on the airsickness bag in my lap.

I'd obviously learned about anxiety in medical school, but I wasn't prepared to experience it firsthand. Anxiety happened to other people. It was the purview of mousy, waifish, ninety-year-old ladies who walked their surly puppies in my neighborhood every morning—not me.

That September 14 flight unleashed a panic in me that, once freed, proved unrelenting. Every flight became a terror. On a particularly turbulent flight, my seatmate, an older man who'd been a stranger when we boarded, had to talk me through implacable tears. I needed to get off, but I had no place to go.

And then the panic metastasized. At a small-group Bible study later that year, I had to read aloud a passage from an Old Testament prophet. Ezekiel describes a valley of dry human bones that knit themselves together into skeletons, and then wrap themselves in sinew, tendon, muscle, and skin while he watches. As these dry bones came to life, I died. Tightness, tremulousness, palpitations, shortness of breath—I ran to the bathroom to hide. Soon every public speaking event became another chance for panic to remind me that it controlled me.

ANXIETY PLAGUES ME WHEN I can't get away. I don't get anxious on trains because trains stop. There's an out. I don't get anxious in a car because I'm in control.

But planes? I'm stuck in a metal tube for a predetermined time, with zero options and with four hundred eyes waiting for me to mess up. If I don't keep it together, everyone will notice the guy in the aisle seat having a panic attack. I'll prove to the world—again—that I'm a failure.

A quarter of Americans experience a panic attack at some point in their lives;[5] generalized anxiety afflicts about 5 percent.[6] And anxiety is as irrational as it is common. Over the next fifteen years, I became adept at reading turbulence maps, weather reports, and seat configurations, hoping that knowing where turbulence would happen and how the fuselage would react could blunt the panic.

But I couldn't reason myself into calm. I tried: I know the stats. I know flying is mind-bogglingly safe. In the nine years and one hundred million commercial flights before April 2018, the United States had *zero* air-related fatalities.[7] The chance of dying in an airplane crash is on the order of one in ten million. I'd need to fly every day for thirteen thousand years before I'd be expected to die in a plane crash, on average.

But logic couldn't convince me out of panic attacks, nor does it work for any of the 6.5 percent of Americans who fear flying.[8] Of the two hundred people in a plane with me, at least a dozen others are just as freaked out, just as sure that they're going to fail to keep it all together. The specifics may vary—turbulence terrifies me; others worry about hijackings, or throwing up on their neighbors, or a bird strike to the engines, or having to pee when the seat belt sign is on—but the constricted chest and rapid breathing feel the same.

Because I couldn't reason myself out of panic, it started to reason with me—and it wasn't kind. How, it asked, did I think I could work in global health if I couldn't even fly without a panic attack? How would I speak about Alimou and Andrew and the 143 million others who don't get the surgery they need every year, if standing on a stage, staring into the darkness beyond the spotlights, feels like bungee jumping without a rope?

Had I really solved for why if the solution meant paralyzing panic attacks? Anytime I thought I had, panic was there, patting me on the head. "Bless your little heart," it said. "Aren't you just *adorable*, thinking you can actually accomplish all that?"

IT'S BEEN TWO DECADES since that September 14 flight. I'm no longer afraid of flying.

Don't get me wrong—I still find flying miserable. Herded through nylon cordons and metal stanchions, flesh pressed against servile flesh, under the unfazed eyes of airline employees who want to be there about as much as we do, we're folded into metal tubes, wedged into seats assigned like they were on the *Titanic*, and offered ten-dollar snack boxes. Flying is wretched. But it no longer scares me.

In the decade and a half that it took me to be able to write that, panic taught me a counterintuitive—and crucial—lesson about itself: to become unafraid of flying, I had to be afraid of flying. To make peace with panic, I had to submit to panic.

It wasn't a lesson I learned easily. I spent the first fourteen years trying to make the panic go away. I visited psychologists who wanted to trace the anxiety to my parents and to the strictures of an all-boys Catholic school. I talked to hypnotists, life coaches, and faith healers. I read books written by pilots and flight attendants. I bought a flight simulator and played it every night for six months. I joined focus groups, support groups, internet groups, and prayer groups. Finally, I turned to drugs.

Benzodiazepines are among the most widely prescribed medications in the United States.[9] Because they work in concert with an inhibitory neurotransmitter called gamma-aminobutyric acid (or GABA), they're mind-altering drugs by design.

GABA keeps our neurons from overactivity. It works by attaching itself to specific neuronal receptor proteins, and, once attached, by changing the neurons' inner workings. It increases the threshold at which these neurons fire, thereby stabilizing them and making them less likely to send a signal. Without GABA, we'd be tetanic balls of tension.

Benzodiazepines like Ativan and Xanax accentuate GABA's

inhibitory effect, prolonging the neuronal changes it creates. As a result, benzodiazepines are great sedatives. They can also cause mood swings, euphoria, and occasional erratic behavior.

I became familiar with both the sedation and the mood swings. Anytime I took an Ativan, I'd feel a soft wash of euphoria almost immediately. When it wore off, however, I'd crash into a predictably deep sadness. I learned to warn loved ones to disregard anything I said while I was under the drug's influence.

I hated Ativan, but because it was the only thing that blunted the panic attacks, I figured that solving for why just meant a life of transatlantic flights swaddled in temporary, medicated euphoria, followed by the inevitable, irritable, teary crash.

DOCTORS HAVE AN ARSENAL of treatments for anxiety, of which anxiolytics like Ativan are not the first line. Other drugs like Zoloft—which is not a benzodiazepine—can be as effective without the crash.

And there are hundreds of nonpharmacological techniques that claim to make anxiety disappear—some of which have serious science behind them. Solid randomized, controlled trials, for example, have shown that breathing exercises can decrease feelings of tension and anxiety.[10] Breathing practitioners swear by their specific breathing techniques. I'm personally a fan of box breathing: you breathe in for four seconds, hold it for four seconds, breathe out for four, and then hold for four again.[11]

There's also evidence for things like a mindfulness practice,[12] cannabidiol,[13] or cognitive behavioral therapy with applied relaxation techniques.[14] I've tried them all.

But here's what I've found: none of them makes the anxiety disappear. At most, these techniques only blunt it.

What worked for me is exposure. Exposure therapy is one of the oldest treatments around, and it remains among the most effective. A fascinating 2001 study in the *British Journal of Psychiatry* compared Zoloft alone, repeated trigger exposure, or both, for patients with anxiety. Initially, the drug won. It performed far better than exposure therapy.[15]

But that was only in the short term. Zoloft's effects didn't hold, and a year later the results flipped. Only patients who underwent exposure therapy, by itself, showed sustained improvement. Zoloft-treated patients actually got worse, as did those who got both Zoloft and exposure therapy.[16]

Look, I'm not a psychiatrist. Don't take these paragraphs as medical advice. It's probably a good rule not to take psychiatric advice from a surgeon anyway.

If you struggle with anxiety, your treatment plan should be made in conjunction with your physician. Especially if you use medications like benzodiazepines, do *not* alter your medication regimen without a professional. Withdrawal from these drugs can be lethal.

I may not be able to give you psychiatric advice, but what I can do is speak to my own experience. The fundamental problem with my original approach to anxiety—and the fundamental problem with how most of us approach difficult emotions—is that I viewed it as something to overcome, something to shut down. I wanted a life without anxiety. But to experience no anxiety is to be inhuman.

Psychologist Steven Hayes has demonstrated that attempting to avoid painful feelings like anxiety only serves to strengthen them. He likens these feelings to Dostoyevsky's polar bear: "Try," the Russian author once wrote, "not to think of a polar bear, and you will see that the cursed thing will come to mind every minute."[17]

Instead of running from anxiety, trying to force it to go away, or trying to set up a life that avoids it, Hayes recommends complete submission to it. He recommends accepting painful feelings like anxiety—even being willing to be overcome by them—and acting in line with your values anyway.

In fact, he thinks these painful feelings are signposts. Just like failure is a harbinger of *yet*, the painful feelings we try to avoid may be harbingers of *why*. As an example, Hayes presents a patient with social anxiety. "Very likely," he writes, "this is a person who values connections with others. If connecting with others was not of any importance, the person would not be socially phobic."

The painful feelings we try avoid, like anxiety, are subconscious way-markers, pointing us toward our why. "In our pain," he writes, "we are given some guidance toward our values."[18]

And, as we push toward our values, we also push right into the pain. Living a life according to your values won't make anxiety go away. In fact, like it does with failure, it'll force you to confront it head-on. "In our values," Hayes concludes, "we find our pain."

He's right. I wanted so terribly not to be anxious about flying because I wanted so terribly to work in global surgery. That was how I planned to live out my values. I thought I needed to overcome the anxiety before I could commit to this path.

But that's not true. I needed, instead, to commit anyway. I needed to make scary decisions about my why, *despite* the anxiety. I needed to be intentional about putting anxiety in its place, about reminding it that my values superseded it, and not the other way around.

To do so, I needed to turn the willingness dial—to borrow Hayes's image—all the way up. I had to be prepared to have panic attacks on planes so that I could learn that these panic attacks were powerless when they were pitted against my values.

I started exposing myself to panic without Ativan. Instead of trying everything I could to make the anxiety disappear, I submitted to its heavy hand. Besides, I'd grown tired of the post-euphoria crash.

My first nonmedicated flight showed me anxiety's primary weakness: panic attacks don't last. If I was willing to let them come, then they'd always leave. Panic was temporary, and that made it powerless. The day I made my first, short, Ativan-less flight, the person next to me again saw tears. Only this time, they weren't tears of panic. They were tears of redemption.

After that, the dominoes fell quickly. Less than a year after my first unmedicated flight, I flew from Boston to Adelaide, Australia—forty-eight hours of travel—without any medications. Getting over the panic took two things: it took exposure, and it took accepting the panic and choosing to act in line with my values anyway.

YOUR ANXIETY MAY NOT manifest as diagnosable panic attacks, but it will be there once you leave the moving sidewalk. The world outside is out of your control, and that's terrifying.

Anxiety is a scoundrel that plagues the road to why. Instead of avoiding it or trying to silence it, experiment with turning the willingness dial all the way up. Don't cross your fingers and screw your eyes shut and pretend that fear isn't there. Don't wait until it's gone, because it'll never be gone. To quote Brené Brown one last time, "You can choose courage or you can choose comfort....You cannot have both."[19]

Don't wait to jump off the moving sidewalk until it's safe. Jump, despite the panic. In fact, jump straight into the panic. "The impediment to action advances action," wrote Marcus Aurelius in *Meditations*. "What stands in the way becomes the way."[20]

Welcome the anxiety. Say to that scoundrel, "I acknowledge you. You're here. I'm scared. Now what do I have to do to live according to my values anyway?"

On the days I do that, anxiety loses its power.

Chapter 19

———⚓———

You are never dedicated to something you have complete confidence in.

—ROBERT M. PIRSIG

EVERY TIME I'M ON the hospital ship, there's one patient whose case makes me lose sleep. In 2016, Houefassi was that patient.

Days are long on the *Africa Mercy*, but the weeks are short. From seven o'clock in the morning to six o'clock in the evening, we shuttle nonstop through operating rooms, admission clinics, outpatient clinics, screening clinics, radiology, pharmacy, laboratory, and wards with fifteen to twenty patients. Five operative days a week, our scalpels beat back a deluge of tumors grown too big for their hosts. I'm most immersed in my why when I'm working as a surgeon in West Africa. I'm most at my center when my heart is turned toward the poor.

Despite the routine, however, there's always a patient who breaks it, always one whose tumor feels just wrong, whose anatomy strays, whose scans betray more extensive disease than the physical exam suggests.

For thirty-six-year-old Houefassi, the tumor grew from the

root of her left neck. She faced the same access barriers Alimou faced, the same ones that keep over 90 percent of the African continent's population from getting surgery. Too few patients present for care while their tumors are still small.

But there's big, and there's Houefassi big.

Her tumor engulfed normal structures in her neck, pushing her carotid artery backward against her spine and enveloping her jugular vein altogether. Like an occupying force, it expanded unimpeded, asserting its dominance over all the anatomy between her esophagus and her skin. The vagus nerve, which controls crucial functions like breathing, speaking, and a regular heartbeat, lay somewhere between the tumor and the spine. Other nerves that controlled Houefassi's shoulder, her diaphragm, her tongue, and how she moved her face had been displaced by this invader's claims of sovereignty.

Radiographically, I could see the culprit: a small thyroid mass, plastered against Houefassi's trachea, had sent its neoplastic settlers throughout her left neck.

I didn't sleep well for days before Houefassi's operation. Sometimes, cases that make me lose sleep end up being easier than their scans suggest. Maybe it's because those scans drive me back to the textbooks to pore over anatomy I've spent a career navigating. Maybe it's because I stay up visualizing how the tumor and its vasculature relate, planning what I'll do if I can't free the mass, and plotting exit strategies should things get too hoary. Sometimes these cases end up being easy.

Sometimes they don't.

I was nervous the morning of Houefassi's case. Since I'd once read that the act of chewing releases serotonin—and that serotonin keeps the brain from getting too anxious[1]—I chew gum when I'm nervous. I'd bought a new pack in preparation for her operation.

As I scrubbed, all I could see were the risks she and I were taking. I saw Houefassi bleeding. I saw an unresectable tumor. I saw the extended conversation we'd have the next morning, the one where I explained to her why she woke up with a noose-like incision in her neck, overlying a tumor I never took out.

Before I even put knife to skin, I doubted I could help Houefassi.

IF ANXIETY IS A rapscallion plaguing the road to why, then doubt is its twittering travel buddy. They're inseparable; you'll meet them both as soon as you leave the moving sidewalk.

But we don't talk very much about doubt. We enjoy doubt about as much as we enjoy taking a cold shower with our clothes on. In response, perhaps, to the uncertainty of our modern public discourse, an insidiously toxic positivity infiltrates our worldview and banishes doubt.

That's not altogether unreasonable either: studies demonstrate a persistent, significant correlation between doubt and performance among athletes.[2] Scientists have studied motivational self-talk (things like "I can do it," "Let's go," or "Give it your all") since at least the 1980s. Back then, Brent Rushall and Maureen Shewchuk showed that positive self-talk led to statistically significant improvements in swimming performance.[3] Twenty years later, Antonis Hatzigeorgiadis and his colleagues at the University of Thessaly combined data from thirty-two studies of 2,741 athletes to show that positive self-talk works across many unrelated athletic disciplines.[4]

The canonical example of the power of positive self-talk

happened on February 22, 1980. The United States Olympic hockey team faced the Soviet Union in a medal-round game. The odds were stacked against the amateur American team, especially because the mostly-pro Russian team had won gold in five out of the prior six Olympic Games. The Russian goalkeeper, Vladislav Tretiak, was widely recognized as the best in the world.

In the locker room before the game, Herb Brooks, the American coach, told his team: "You were born to be a player. You were meant to be here. This moment is yours."[5] In what became known as the Miracle on Ice, the American team broke a 3–3 tie in the final ten seconds of the game to capture gold.

I was five when the Miracle on Ice happened, and I remember it. It was that electric. In it, we saw the quintessential American story: the underdog's victory and the power of belief. In an interview afterwards, Brooks admitted, "It's kind of corny and I could see them thinking, 'Here goes Herb again....' But I believed it."[6]

Athletes who doubt themselves, like I did in Cincinnati, consistently perform worse than those who believe they belong on the field—even against the evidence. Those who "fake it till they make it" outperform better-trained athletes whose minds convince them they never should have been on the starting block in the first place.

Just as Herb's words—"You were meant to be here. This moment is yours"—carried historical force, their opposite can be just as powerful. A friend and fellow ninja warrior is, hands down, one of the strongest people I know. He can hold himself in a one-armed pull-up forever. His endurance is infinite. Away from competition, he's got mind-blowing strength.

But he enters every competition expecting to fail. His

self-talk fixates on the specific ways each competitor will out-perform him. And his performance in competition never comes close to reflecting his strength—because he talks himself out of it. It's as if Herb Brooks's doppelgänger sits on his right shoulder: "You're *not* supposed to be here," it whispers. "You *weren't* born for this. This moment *isn't* yours."

His doubt is kryptonite.

STORIES LIKE THESE, BACKED by decades of science, strongly implicate positivity in performance. I'd be hypocritical to deny that. However, an exclusionary embrace of positivity and cat-egorical denial of doubt quickly turn toxic.

The American workplace is a prime example of this toxic positivity. Our offices are grindingly cheery: if we say yes, stay upbeat, and don't question authority, we rise. On the other hand, we doubt at our own peril.

Julie Donley, author of *The Journey Called YOU*, instructs her readers, "You want people to feel good after being in your presence."[7] Above all else, the mantra is "Stay positive. Don't rock the boat. Follow the leader, no matter what."

Any employee who threatens this positivity with skepticism and doubt risks being labeled confrontational, and confronta-tional employees are problem employees. Being a good worker often has less to do with productivity than it does with staying optimistic and suppressing doubt.

If you come from a traditional religious background like I do, you're also intimately familiar with this suppression of doubt. In many religious communities, doubt is an impos-tor to be routed, a Benedict Arnold to be tried and executed. "For centuries now our culture has cultivated the idea that the *skeptical* person is always smarter than one who believes. You can almost be as stupid as a cabbage as long as you *doubt*," the theologian Dallas Willard disparaged in *Hearing God*.[8]

I have sat at the feet of countless preachers who cast doubt as an enemy and the believer as an armored defender of the faith. I've been instructed to kill doubt before it kills me. In the words of Greg Laurie, doubt is often perceived as "an act of spiritual treason."[9] These preachers use metaphors of war, of bloodshed, and—terrifyingly to the doubter—of final, eternal defeat.

David Jeremiah, for example, writes, "There's a battle for your faith going on right now.... Too much doubt, disillusionment, and discouragement—and you'll give up.... If you find yourself defeated in this battle, Satan receives the glory."[10]

Oof. Once doubt is permitted, then the Prince of Darkness himself gets the glory. Doubt, Jeremiah implies, must be fought with all our might, lest Beelzebub capture our very souls. This stance brooks no discussion: if we don't get the doubt behind us, we might as well take Dante's *Inferno* as a travel guide.

It's immaterial to preachers like this that doubt is an inevitable part of the human experience. To them, skepticism is anathema, nothing more than a tine in Satan's red pitchfork. Though I'm convinced theirs is an ultimately untenable position, it has alluring power. Because doubt is so uncomfortable, a hard-line stance that rejects it altogether feels protective.

Not all evangelicals grow up as dogmatic as I did, for sure. But even for gentler adherents, doubt can never be more than a way station, a rest stop on the road to absolute fealty. It must stay ephemeral, because stopping at doubt opens the door to the devil. Chuck Swindoll has reportedly said, "It is the right of every believer to go *through* halls of doubt *on their way to rooms of truth*."[11]

*   *   *

IN WORK, IN SPORTS, in religion, we strive to stamp out doubt wherever we find it. We try to subjugate skepticism to the idolatry of a kept peace, or to the worship of absolutes.

Susan David, a Harvard psychologist, calls this *the tyranny of positivity*. "Being positive," she says, "has become a new form of moral correctness.... It's cruel. Unkind. And ineffective. And we do it to ourselves, and we do it to others."[12]

It's also counterproductive. Toxic positivity eventually amplifies doubt and negativity. In the same way that trying to make anxiety go away strengthens anxiety's hold, pretending doubt doesn't exist gives it more power. "You might think you're in control of unwanted emotions when you ignore them," Dr. David says. "But in fact, they control you." Doubt always appears. Always.

That's because doubt is ubiquitous. We haven't stamped it out in hundreds of years of trying, because we simply can't. It's not just a way station—it's an ever-present companion, especially once we leave the moving sidewalk. "Doubt," writes Thomas Merton, "is by no means opposed to genuine faith, but it mercilessly examines and questions the spurious 'faith' of everyday life, the human faith which is nothing but passive acceptance of conventional opinion."[13]

Doubt won't go away when preachers stridently deny it, nor does it shirk when bosses minimize it. It doesn't disappear through calls to unquestioned fealty or hide from toxic positivity.

So instead of trying to stamp it out, experiment with welcoming it. Try encouraging it. And at the same time, doubt it.

DOUBT WILL SURPRISE YOU with both its tenacity and its perfect timing. Especially amid inevitable failure, it'll be the loudest voice in your mental chorus. It'll be the audience member throwing tomatoes. It'll be your fiercest competitor at the starting block, the one you viscerally know is better than you.

Since you can't escape doubt, stop trying. Doubt has a role in our mental chorus: it softens failures and promotes preparation. At its worst, it argues that if we never allow ourselves to believe in success, then *when* we fail, disappointment won't hurt as much. Of course we failed! We knew we weren't capable from the outset. The sports psychologist Jim Afremow calls this a *fear of winning*.

Left unchecked, this defense mechanism is maladaptive. Properly held, however, it can be helpful, because positivity alone cannot replace preparation.[14] Not even Herb Brooks could completely overcome a lack of training. Just believing I could take out Houefassi's tumor would never have guided my scalpel well enough.

At its best, then, doubt encourages a grind. Putting our heads down and working, day in and day out, is a stronger predictor of success than simply psyching ourselves up.

When I first began public speaking, I would spend actual months preparing for a single talk. I would slog through the talk, practicing it three times a day, every day, until it became so ingrained in my muscles that I knew exactly when I'd take each breath. I had to turn down speaking engagements if they were less than two months away, because I didn't have enough time to prepare.

I reasoned that, if I'd been invited onstage to play a Bach concerto, then I'd deserve all the boos if I hadn't practiced. Why should public speaking be any different? I've gotten a bit better—I no longer need to know where I'm going to take each breath, and I'm more comfortable ad-libbing parts of a talk—but a persistent doubt about my public speaking abilities continues to ensure that I'm as prepared as possible when I get onstage. I still practice my talks like Joshua Bell practices Mozart.

Doubt that leads to preparation isn't a rapscallion. It's a friend. Welcome it.

AND ALSO DOUBT IT. Doubt your doubt.

Susan David advocates emotional agility instead of the tyranny of positivity. "Radical acceptance of all of our emotions—even the messy, difficult ones—is the cornerstone to resilience, thriving, and true, authentic happiness."[15]

Our mental chorus doesn't sing in unison. Behind the tenor of doubt is the bass reminding us that we *are* the smart, successful, strong, and emotionally stable people we hope we might be. Under the soloist who warbles our mediocrity lie the harmonies of our successes.

Half a century ago, John Gottman and Robert Levenson undertook a decade-long longitudinal study of couples. Their findings first introduced the dogma that it takes five positive interactions to counteract a single negative one.[16] What they found in marriage relationships is also true of the only relationship we can never leave—the one with ourselves.

We treat ourselves like Gottman and Levenson's couples: one failure weighs five times more than one success. We brood on a misstep for days, while a win lasts minutes before we're off to the next goal. We listen to the soloists, and we ignore the chorus behind them.

Logically, there's no reason we should act this way. We've failed and we've succeeded. We have evidence that both the tenor and the bass sing the truth. We only hear one voice more clearly because we choose to. We cultivate a fantastically well-developed long-term memory for failure—and a fantastically underdeveloped long-term memory for success.

In other words, we take doubt at its word.

Instead, find the middle path. Welcome doubt, encourage it, and also doubt it. The loudest voices in your chorus aren't infallible—they're just loud. They've been wrong before, and they'll be wrong again. Theirs is a skewed view of you.

Instead of silencing them, use them to motivate you to prepare. And also force them to sing in harmony with all the other voices that remind you of the times you've succeeded. The most emotionally agile people, Dr. David found, are those whose relationship with their emotions is balanced. Solving for why demands this precarious balance. It insists on a radical acceptance of doubt, on using that doubt to drive your grind, and on simultaneously doubting the assertions it makes.

HOUEFASSI'S CASE WAS HARD. Really hard.

And doubt did its job: it forced me to prepare. Her case went as badly as my Hitchcockian nightmares had predicted. Everything bled. Clots covered my hands, my gown, my shoes, and my mask. If I brushed a gauze sponge across anything in her neck, it bled. If I cauterized it, it bled. If I cauterized next to it, it bled. If I thought about cauterizing it, it bled. If I lifted it, moved it, set it back, looked at it—it still bled.

Advancing millimeters at a time, I had to peel the tumor away from the anatomy that made Houefassi function—the nerves that moved her shoulder and her diaphragm, the vessels that supplied her face and her brain—all while her blood pooled around my shoes and the anesthesia machine beeped in time with her heart.

And the whole thing was on camera. For six months, an Australian film crew had been on board, getting footage for what would turn into an eight-episode National Geographic series. They met Houefassi and her bulbous tumor in the screening line. "She's it," they said. "We want an episode about her."

In the back right corner of the operating room that day, at a safe distance from the blood, sat the director, his soundman, and their unforgiving, gunmetal paraphernalia. I was miked. There would be no cursing.

I'd booked the case for three hours. Six hours in, we began to sound like a family road trip. "How much longer," the director asked. "Not far now," I said.

Nine hours—and five units of blood—after my knife first broke skin, Houefassi was tumor-free. Every hazard that doubt had prepared me for had happened. In addition to the blood, she lost a jugular vein that was completely encased in the tumor.* Everything else remained intact. Her shoulder moved. Her face worked. Her heart beat regularly. Her brain still got oxygen. And she left the hospital a few days later.

All because of doubt.

---

* You can survive without one of your jugular veins. The jugular vein on the other side—as well as other collateral vessels—quickly picks up the slack. It's one of the beautiful things about operating in the head and neck: the body has a sophisticated network of collateral vasculature, overlapping safety nets that keep blood going to the important bits.

Chapter 20

A man knows when he has found his vocation when he stops thinking about how to live and begins to live.

—THOMAS MERTON

IN MARCH OF 2020, I performed my 2,500th procedure since finishing surgical training. His name was Lamine. He first presented to Mercy Ships without a nose.

The problem started when he was one, or when he was six, or when he was eight. He gave a different story every time you asked. At twenty-four, however, he'd lived with it for most of his life.

The problem is called noma, and it's a disease you've almost certainly never seen before. That's because, outside of resource-constrained countries, only isolated cases—like a child during the start of the HIV epidemic[1]—have occurred since the concentration camps of World War II.[2]

Noma is fundamentally a disease of poverty, malnutrition, and suppressed immune systems. It exists primarily in countries bordering the Sahara and, far less frequently, in poorer areas of Asia. Only 10 to 20 percent of noma patients survive. Of those who do, most lose their faces.

Literally.

The disease begins with an inciting event in a child—classically a viral infection like measles or chicken pox—superimposed on a backdrop of malnutrition and poor oral hygiene. In patients who survive the inciting viral infection, normal bacteria living in their mouths and noses overpower an immune system weakened by the virus. Unchecked, these tiny commensal organisms start feeding on the flesh of the patient's face. Symptoms can be as mild as bleeding gums and bad breath—or as severe as Lamine's.

His commensal bacteria had stolen his entire upper lip, all of his nose, and the vision in his left eye. His left lower eyelid had scarred down to the corner of his mouth, and where the eyeball used to be, he was left with a fibrotic, sightless globe. A crater sat in the middle of his face, connecting the outside world to his throat. He covered it with a head wrap.

Fixing Lamine's face took a three-surgeon marathon: Gary Parker, me, and an Australian plastic surgeon named David Chong. We removed the scarred eyeball and replaced it with a prosthesis, excised his lower eyelid, borrowed tissue from his forehead to create a new nose, flipped part of his tongue upward to close the opening where his hard palate had been, shifted some of his cheek forward, and then rotated both ends of his lower lip superiorly to fashion a new, but smaller, upper lip. These borrowed tissues obstructed his natural airway, so he also got a tracheotomy tube in his neck to help him breathe, and a second tube to connect his esophagus to liquid nutrition with which we'd feed him for the next three weeks.

A surgery like Lamine's requires follow-up procedures. The rotational flaps that turn a forehead into a nose, or that move the tongue to the roof of the mouth, have to be released a few weeks later. The tracheotomy tube must be removed. And the tiny mouth opening has to be widened. Lamine's care takes meticulous follow-up and small, planned (and sometimes unplanned) revision operations.

And they're all routine.

In a decade and a half of working in sub-Saharan African countries, I've done nearly three hundred procedures on noma patients. I've performed hundreds of tracheotomies in my career, hundreds of skin grafts, dozens of rotational flaps. I've taken out one hundred fifty jaw tumors like the one Alimou had. I've treated scores of African patients with albinism like Andrew. These operations are my routine.

OUTSIDE OF WHY, I spent monumental amounts of energy thinking about how to live, how to survive, how to wake up every morning, how to repeat each day—and monumental amounts of energy thinking about how to escape that routine. The Gary Parker Rule showed me drudgery, banality, and the mundane pursuit of privilege. I saw an endless train of tracheotomies, multitudes of mandibulectomies, and infinite flaps, stretching out over thirty years.

And it was soul crushing.

You, too, may see all of these. Or you may see ceaseless emails, meetings, commutes, and trips. Or diaper changes, three-year-old tantrums, sullen teenagers, and finally the loneliness of an empty nest.

Outside of why, our days fuse into dreary, unremarkable

discontent, so it's tempting to blame that discontent on the routines themselves. It feels like their mundanity is killing us.

But that's the tail wagging the dog. Every career involves monotony, every path its drudgery. Every journey is repetitive. This was Steve Lacey's lesson to the thirteen wide-eyed medical students coming home from a mission trip in Mexico.

Whether it's writing two thousand words a day, doing six more tonsillectomies, getting to inbox zero, rehearsing our lines, recording the next podcast, making the next trade, taking the same train, driving the same road, or seeing the next Lamine, life is composed of routines.

In fact, someone out there pines after yours. To a paramedic, for example, there's little glamorous about his hundredth call to pick up a drunk college student. To you and me, a ride-along on an ambulance sounds thrilling. I asked Dave Cavanagh, a friend, Boston-area firefighter, and ninja athlete, to describe his job. He wrote: "We do the same chores every day, at the same time: washing the trucks, sweeping the floor, and overall basic janitorial things. I busted my butt to get this job, and I spend more time cleaning up after grown men in the firehouse than I do actually helping people. It's mind-numbing, really."

THE PROBLEM WITH FIXATING on routine as the *cause* of our dissatisfaction is that it's not the primary culprit. We're often tempted to shake things up as some sort of iconoclastic rebellion against the jails that we find ourselves in, but this misses the point: dynamiting our routines leads to imprudence far more often than it leads to epiphany.

Routine, instead, serves one of two purposes. It's either how we numb ourselves while we're on the moving sidewalk, or it's the grind with which we embody our why. Because it's often the former, we indict the routine and its monotony, blind to the fact that the true criminal is the moving sidewalk itself. The solution to our ennui doesn't lie in the pursuit of the new for the sake of the new. It lies in getting off the moving sidewalk.

I still see an endless train of tracheotomies, multitudes of mandibulectomies, and infinite flaps, stretching out over decades. Jaw tumors like Alimou's and rotational flaps like the ones we used on Lamine—these operations are my bread and butter in West Africa. They're also the same operations I did before I left my Boston practice. I rotated the same flaps, reconstructed the same defects, went through the same operative steps, and followed the same procedures as I do now.

Back then, I sought excitement to counteract the boredom. But no sneaky trip to Atlantic City, no card game with Russian soldiers, and no new experience had the power to break the dissatisfaction.

Solving for why hasn't made life any less routine. The difference, however, is obvious: routine was once the anesthetic I used to numb myself to the moving sidewalk. Now, it is the how with which I live out my why.

Don't search for the solution to your ennui in new experiences—you'll face those soon enough. Instead, as with anxiety and with doubt, view the boredom as a check-engine light telling you that something's wrong. What, exactly, may not yet be clear, but the niggling dissatisfaction you feel in your routine means you need to pause and to diagnose. And eventually, it means you'll need to make systematic, intentional decisions that turn you toward your values, decisions like those guided by the Gary Parker Rule.

For me, the solution to the dissatisfaction meant quitting my practice altogether; for you it's going to mean something else. But whatever it means, it'll be confusing, at least initially. It'll force you to face the terrors I've spent the last few chapters talking about: anxiety, doubt, and failure. It'll require exploration, construction, crucifixion, and resurrection.

And in the end, it'll lead you to beauty. To wonder. And to worship. And that's how I want to finish this book.

Chapter 21

⎯⎯ ᴧ ⎯⎯

*Remember to look up at the stars and not down at
your feet.*

—STEPHEN HAWKING

SHE WORE A GOLD-LINED, forest-green sari. Her hair was
wound in a bun; stray, graying wisps framed her small face.
Her shoes were the expensive kind, as was the jewelry around
her wrist. In a warren of pedestrian alleys behind Varanasi's
kaleidoscopic buildings, she crouched over the curb.

My mind refused to parse what she had done until she
stood up, retrieved a plastic bottle from the brocaded clutch
in her left armpit, and sprinkled its water on her backside. In
one practiced motion, she shimmied the sari down, replaced
the makeshift bidet in her purse, and finished her morning
constitutional.

Varanasi is a vertiginous windmill of color, burning bodies,
and the crush of 1.2 million people living in a city half the size
of Philadelphia. It's ancient. It was founded at the same time as
King David's ascension to Israel's throne, the arrival of the Lat-
ins on the Italian peninsula, and the invention of the alphabet

by the Phoenicians. Hindu pilgrims travel to Varanasi for high holy days and to bury their dead in India's most important river.

Varanasi is also boisterously dirty. In its alleys, humanity jostles for space with stores, hostels, temples, and sacred cattle. Lassi hawkers ply their tangy wares from road edges, their yogurt drinks peppered with dirt and diesel.

I visited Varanasi in 2007, one stop on that six-month journey from Iceland to New Zealand. I've experienced nothing in my life quite as wondrous, overwhelming, nauseating, exhilarating, and horrifying as travel in India, especially by train.

Most Indian trains have three service classes. In third class, seats aren't assigned. Boarding means trusting your body to the fluid dynamics of crowds, hoping they carry you into the car.

In second class, seats are mostly assigned, but that doesn't stop the pre-arrival scrum of passengers leaping aboard a still-moving train. First-class passengers get a cabin to themselves and a few six-legged refugees.

In 2007, second-class berths on overnight trains were purposely oversold, much like airline flights are today. Unlike airlines, which can't fit two passengers into a single seat, the Indian rail system will transport all ticketed passengers who show up, even if that means an overcrowded car. To accomplish this, the rail company designates some berths as half beds. There's no way for the novice Indian rail rider to know which berths these are. They don't cost any less than full-berth tickets. They just exist. And if the other ticket holder for a half berth shows up, as I experienced on the overnight train into Varanasi, then both passengers spend an uncomfortable night in stony silence, toes against the other person's ears.

*   *   *

THERE ARE TWO WAYS to approach Varanasi, two ways to see this dizzying Indian city. Varanasi can be mud, or it can be color. Its visitors can be distracted by the dirt, or they can see the brilliant tableau that rises around them. They can focus on the open defecation, the gastroenteritis, and the cow manure. Or they can marvel at the gilded green saris, the brocaded clutches, and the dance of thirty separate spices married with heaps of brightly colored vegetables surrounding a glistening white scoop of rice.

Jumping off the moving sidewalk is like taking a train into Varanasi. We're offered the Varanasi choice: focus on failures, doubts, anxieties, and routine, or find wonder. They're both there—the wonder and the failure. One keeps us awed; the other keeps us cowed. One makes the leap off the moving sidewalk worth it; the other just makes us want to run back to safety.

Our first steps off the moving sidewalk are always uncertain. Hyper-attuned to what we're leaving—to what could be and what could have been and what could go wrong—we feel a perilous tension. Like the grapes that Tantalus could never reach, these steps make us acutely aware of both the beauty that awaits us where we want to go and the distance between that beauty and where we are now. If you're anything like me, that'll feel like the dust and the grime of Varanasi, and not like the spices of a thali.

THE SOLUTION TO THIS tension is hopeful wonder, something the ethos of Work has beaten out of us.

While it's true that we spend less physical time at work

than in prior generations—on average, about five hours fewer per week than in the 1950s[1]—we're still bound to the ethos of Work.

We know it's unhealthy, so we concoct solutions by changing the structure of work itself. For example, Google's employees famously spend 20 percent of their time working on personal projects that are supposed to benefit Google.[2] The American Bar Association encourages lawyers to "render at least fifty hours of pro bono legal services per year,"[3] often in fields outside of their primary practice. And in 2020, Finland's prime minister called for a six-hour workday and a four-day workweek.[4]

Although there is evidence to suggest that shorter workweeks do improve employee productivity, that's just a gilded lily: finding the cure to the ethos of Work in things that improve productivity is still the ethos of Work.

Indeed, fewer than 10 percent of Google employees actually take advantage of their 20 percent time, and while four in five lawyers believe that pro bono work is important, only half actually do it because they're all simply too busy.

Work has become a kind of worship, the "kind of worship you just gradually slip into, day after day . . . without ever being fully aware that that's what you're doing," in the words of David Foster Wallace.[5]

In the 1930s, the British macroeconomist John Maynard Keynes predicted that, by the twenty-first century, "for the first time since creation, man will be faced with his real, permanent problem—how to occupy leisure."[6] He was prescient: we've spent so much time subject to the ethos of Work that we've forgotten how to occupy leisure. Even though we desperately need hopeful wonder to keep us from running back to the moving sidewalk, we don't know how to create it. Instead, we turn wonder into something suspiciously close to work.

I LEARNED THIS LESSON from a buffalo milk omelet.

Ms. Kaew's wasn't a restaurant you'd seek out. Her establishment had escaped the notice of the on-the-cheap travel guide I'd already carried with me for two weeks in Cambodia in the late 1990s. Like a pretentious New York City speakeasy, her restaurant didn't have a sign out front.

Unlike a pretentious New York City speakeasy, it also didn't have a name.

I doubt her restaurant exists anymore—and if it does, I guarantee I couldn't tell you where in Siem Reap to find it. But the saline aftertaste of Ms. Kaew's buffalo milk omelet still lingers, two and a half decades after I ate it while seated on the dirt floor of her one-room restaurant because its single fuchsia plastic picnic chair was already occupied.

In 2010, Jeroen Nawijn and his colleagues found that people who had taken a vacation in the previous year were significantly happier than those who hadn't.[7] That's right. Someone paid him to study whether vacations make people happier, and, unsurprisingly, they do.

Except, not really.

See, Nawijn found that most vacationers were happier only *prior* to their trips, not after. This led journalists, bloggers, and general philosophizers to twist his counterintuitive conclusions into fantasies about increasing employee satisfaction by permitting them to plan whimsical vacations they'd never actually realize.

Nawijn did, however, find some vacationers who saw a sustained post-trip happiness bump; they remained happy even after they came home. What separates these vacationers from the rest wasn't where they went or how long they spent away. It wasn't what their work structures looked like, or how much free time they got during the day.

It was how they structured the vacation itself. The happiest travelers allowed themselves to wander. They allowed themselves to stop. To experience. To wonder.

Meanwhile, the disgruntled planned. Their vacations were stressful.

In our distinctly modern quest to experience everything, to find the perfect meal, to go on the perfect vacation, to make sure our leisure isn't "wasted," some of us make ourselves *less* happy.

Which brings me back to Ms. Kaew's buffalo milk omelet. I'm one of those disgruntled travelers. If there's anything I'm good at, it's planning. Itineraries make me feel like I'm in control. I like constructing the perfect trip, knowing where I'll sleep every night, picking the restaurants I'll visit, and figuring out exactly how long it'll take me to get from my hostel to the farthest temple on my list.

And sometimes I'm thwarted.

The restaurant I had picked for breakfast in Siem Reap on the morning I met Ms. Kaew had been destroyed. In its place lay a fenced-in hole, one whose future a nearby sign garishly trumpeted: GIVE US ENOUGH TIME AND MONEY, AND WE'LL TURN THIS INAUSPICIOUS PIT INTO AN OVERWROUGHT FIVE-STAR HOTEL!

What the fenced-in hole petulantly refused to do, however, was feed me breakfast.

I'd planned to visit four temples after breakfast that day. I already knew how I'd get from breakfast to the first temple, where I'd have lunch between temples two and three, and where on temple four I'd watch the sunset.

And now, I couldn't even make it to breakfast.

The old man who sat on Ms. Kaew's fuchsia plastic picnic chair ate slate-gray gruel out of a bowl lined with more cracks than the skin on his face. He looked up as I walked by, nodded imperceptibly, and tucked back into his soup.

I hadn't noticed Ms. Kaew's restaurant when I left my hostel that morning. Why would I have? It hadn't made it onto my itinerary, nor had any of the nameless establishments abutting hers in a strip of single-room lean-tos attached by common walls.

Instead, I'd planned to find what the guidebook described as the finest budget breakfast in all of Siem Reap. There was nothing Ms. Kaew or her canteen could offer to match the vaunted authenticity of that restaurant-turned-crater.

I can't tell you why the man's nod pulled me in. All I know is that my gesticulated requests for food were met by a much more perceptible nod from the proprietress. She led me to the right-hand wall of her shop and gestured to the dirt.

"Here," she said. "Breakfast."

I hesitated. I had no idea what breakfast meant to her, but I knew I didn't want any of that gray soup.

After she turned away, I settled against the wall of her lean-to, stretched my legs out, and waited. I'm not going to pretend the waiting was peaceful—it wasn't. It was awkward.

Should I meet the other patron's eyes? He was also eating alone, after all.

Should I take out my book and pretend to read just so I don't look so lonely?

Do I cut and run before it's too late, before a plate appears carrying food I can't describe and tastes my trenchantly Western palate will hate?

He met my eye first. He tipped his spoon at me like an antebellum gentleman tips his hat, a salute, a toast to two men alone at the local. "Just wait," his spoon said. "It'll be worth it."

Make no mistake. The omelet itself wasn't good. Water buffalo milk tastes nothing like the cow milk I was used to, and the cheese that comes from it doesn't either. It's saltier, drier, and gummier.

Curds of it sat atop a rubbery greenish-yellow disc of overcooked eggs, like the nuts in a brownie that no one's willing to admit they dislike. The omelet wasn't good—but it was definitely worth it.

The things I remember from my travels rarely show up in an itinerary. I'm often happiest when I'm thwarted.

I remember chasing down an urchin who nicked my camera as I ate lunch in front of a closed Independence Palace in Saigon. I remember a meal with a rickshaw puller in Thailand, neither of us saying much because neither of us spoke the other's language. And I remember rat kidneys and rice with a pastor and his wife in Liberia.

Those are the ineffable moments that thwarted plans give us. Those are moments of wonder.

On the other hand, the four temples I planned to visit that day? I don't even know if I saw them all. Sure, I remember the grandeur of Angkor Wat and the halcyon sunsets I spent with a sketchbook perched on its walls.

But could I tell you which temple in the complex was which? Could I explain the storied history each hid? Not at all.

They were a box I ticked off, places I visited because I was supposed to, because they were on my itinerary. I saw them. I took pictures I'll never look at again. And I'm no better for it.

The dry buffalo milk omelet I ate while sitting on the dusty floor of a one-table restaurant in Cambodia because the place I'd planned to go was now a hole in the ground. Or feeling the dirt of the restaurant floor under my ragged jeans. Or hearing the proprietress shout directions to her daughter while the latter bent over an open flame. Or the elastic texture of over-cooked eggs with buffalo milk cheese between my teeth.

Those live on.

WE RARELY DISCOVER BUFFALO milk omelets because we ruthlessly plan our vacations to maximize efficiency. We chase the perfect pictures, gathering them like merit badges. We genuflect before experience. But what we don't do is wander. Or wonder.

Instead of wonder, we think the antidote to the ethos of Work is happiness. That's what I—perhaps subconsciously—hoped I'd find once I got off the moving sidewalk. Happiness is etched into our psyches and, at least for Americans, into our founding documents. It's an inalienable right. We're obsessed with it.

Gretchen Rubin wrote her bestselling book *The Happiness Project* after she had an epiphany on a city bus. She decided that a successful life meant a life of happiness.[8] A blog, then the book, then a national movement of people doing happiness projects in happiness groups followed.

The problem is that happiness is evanescent. As an antidote to the ethos of Work, or as something that might keep you from running back to the moving sidewalk, it's frustratingly short-lived. Happiness is a puppy playing fetch, a kitten purring on your lap, a child splashing through puddles. It's what happens at weddings and concerts and amusement parks. It's what we feel when we find a lost sock.

And it doesn't last. As humans, we're nothing if not adaptable. A study of 215 women, all of whom had just been diagnosed with breast cancer, found a bizarre *increase* in their life satisfaction over the two years that followed their cancer diagnosis.[9] This seems initially counterintuitive, but it isn't: these women, like all of us, learned to adapt. They started valuing non-physical quality of life more, while simultaneously devaluing the importance of their physical symptoms.

Adaptability is a spectacular trait. It protects us against pain. It allows us to endure routines—even when they're on the moving sidewalk. But because we're more adaptable to happiness than to pain, adaptability also creates what psychologists call a *hedonic treadmill*.[10] We need more and more happiness to be happy, and when we don't get it, we crash.

The pursuit of happiness isn't unlike addiction. They both work through analogous biochemical pathways. Dopamine, a reward neurotransmitter, hits our brains with a short-term boost of happiness when good things happen.* Seeing the finish line at the end of a race and getting your second wind? That's

---

* Four neurotransmitters are associated with various facets of subjective well-being. Endorphins, released in response to pain, dull the pain and are responsible for things like the runner's high. Oxytocin is involved in interpersonal bonding. It's the "cuddle hormone," released during childbirth, breastfeeding, sex, and even just a hug. Serotonin mediates feelings of significance and belonging. But the hormone most responsible for what we usually call happiness is dopamine.

dopamine. Your first kiss? Dopamine. Finding that lost sock, eating that spectacular meal, or taking the perfect picture? Also dopamine.

The high of cocaine? That's dopamine too.[11] Jeffrey Dahmer's crimes? Dopamine.[12] It's a complex hormone, dopamine, so let's talk about how the body deals with it.

Over millions of years, our bodies have honed a remarkable ability for homeostasis, a balance we maintain through intersecting feedback loops that control our biochemistry and our hormones. Take thyroid hormone, for example. It's secreted from the thyroid gland in the middle of the neck, and it swims through the blood until it finds receptor proteins on distant organs.

When it attaches itself to these receptors, the heart rate increases, the body's core temperature is regulated, and the way we digest food changes, all depending on which organ holds the receptor. These receptors are fine-tuned to respond only to a specific hormone: thyroid receptors respond only to thyroid hormone, estrogen receptors to estrogen, and dopamine receptors to dopamine.

That's how it's supposed to work, at least. When things go awry, however, the body undergoes a complex cellular change,[13] the upshot of which is to protect it against errant hormones. For example, if you have too much thyroid hormone, the receptors for it transform themselves such that they require higher and higher exposure to do their job. Signals that once activated them become insufficient.

In other words, it's as if these receptors lose their metaphorical hearing for a particular signal. This has the consequence it's supposed to: the effects of excess circulating hormone are blunted.

Which brings me back to happiness. Dopamine works in the same way,* and that's bad for happiness. If we pursue happiness as an end to itself, we flood our body with dopamine. This triggers complex biochemical changes, and dopamine receptors lose their hearing. They now require increasing hits to produce the same happiness we once felt, and when we don't get those hits, we feel sadder than we once did.

The pursuit of happiness can never be an antidote to the ethos of Work because we've literally evolved to lose the happiness game. Not only will we never achieve sustained happiness, but it gets harder each time for any one thing to make us happy.

BECAUSE HAPPINESS WON'T KEEP us off the moving sidewalk, solving for why calls for a different antidote to the ethos of Work. It calls for hopeful wonder. It calls for stopping at the buffalo milk omelet, for seeing Varanasi's colors, for feeling the dirt beneath frayed jeans. Specifically, it calls for an awe of the destination you're aiming at and for confident hope that, despite setbacks, you can keep moving toward it.

Creating a life in line with our values does not guarantee happiness. Let me say that again: *Solving for why will not make you happy.* At least, not in the way you think it might. Roy Baumeister's research has shown that, although meaning and happiness intersect, they don't overlap: "a highly meaningful life...is not necessarily a happy one," he and his colleagues write.[14]

But let me assure you, it's a worthwhile one. It's a hopeful,

---

* This is a simplified view of hormones and the process of reward in the brain. Repeated rewards also rewire the brain itself, cementing into our memory the rapid bursts of pleasure associated with these rewards.

wondrous, beautiful life. The road to why is not like a purring kitten or finding a lost sock. It's more like walking through the warren of alleys in Varanasi, with human and bovine excrement at our feet, and riotous color above. It's convoluted and messy. Sometimes it *is* happy, but not always. It's dastardly, and it's slippery.

We could stay on the moving sidewalk, and we'll never have to experience Varanasi's mud in the first place. Once the mud closes around our shoes, however, we must choose whether to see the mud or to look up at the kaleidoscope. We can opt to keep our heads down, and we'll be struck with how much doubt and anxiety and fear we feel.

Or we can focus on the gilded green saris, the brightly colored murals, the smells of the spices, and the bustle of an unknown city. Around every corner on the road to why is meaning. Around every corner is the chance to fail, for sure—but also the chance to discover something we'd never have seen had we stuck to our plan.

Ernest Hemingway once wrote, "Live the full life of the mind, exhilarated by new ideas, intoxicated by the Romance of the unusual."[15] The journey to why can be weird, or it can be intoxicatingly unusual. Instead of looking at the mud, let yourself be transported into hopeful wonder.

Chapter 22

<hr />

Men are what they are because of what they do. Not what they say.

—FREDRIK BACKMAN

At half past ten every Sunday morning, any patient who wants to—and isn't confined to bed—gathers in the pre-op ward on the *Africa Mercy* for church. It's not church like I'm used to. There are no intellectualized, footnoted, culturally relevant sermons delivered by bald men dressed in the casual cool of a blazer and jeans.

This also isn't the church of pressing on, staying positive, never giving up, and claiming the pecuniary blessings of a divine being who exists to provide your SUV with gas and your football team with victories.

It isn't the church you go to for a thing to do on a Sunday morning, for your rock music fix, or for a single hour to cover a multitude of sins.

Ward church is different. It meets in a half-submerged, metal-walled room without windows. Its chairs spill into hallways without windows. Its congregation comes from wards without windows. It's filled with a flock of the transient—volunteers from forty nations, sitting alongside the patients they treat.

And today they dance. The guy on congas? That's Andrew. Two months ago, he had a massive, fungating, mephitic squamous cell carcinoma on his left shoulder. The guy next to him? He almost died in February from a dental infection that had spread to his chest. The men and women dancing, spurring us reserved Westerners to louder singing and syncopated clapping? Their faces are fantastically deformed by Brobdingnagian tumors, scarred expressionless by burns, and bandaged beyond recognition. They jump, shuffle, and shake, with their tracheotomy tubes, their crutches, and their legs casted into immobility. They dance, amputated. They sing, voiceless. They smile, scarred.

This is the church of the outcast, the shunned, the spurned, the Other. This is the congregation of the sideshow. This is my people.

This is worship.

THE GREATEST GIFT ON the road to why is worship.

I started this book by introducing the three pillars of my childhood worldview, the three things I had to unlearn as I solved for why: the ethos of the Other, the ethos of Work, and a childhood faith that lionized absolutes. I've sidled up to the last one throughout this book and then turned away, never actually addressing it.

That's because it was my most fundamental unlearning, and the hardest pillar to get around. It's been the most entrenched; grappling with it hurt. However, death always precedes resurrection, and with resurrection comes worship.

Worship is intensely personal. Maybe you worship the Christian God or the Hebrew God or the Muslim God. Or maybe not. Maybe you're staunchly areligious. Maybe you know better than to worship some sky-being laying down laws about who sleeps with whom. Or maybe you're something in between. Maybe, like the fastest-growing segment of the American population, you're enlightened; you're spiritual but not religious.

No matter which group you identify with, it might feel like a chapter on worship doesn't really apply to you. You're here to solve for why, not to discuss religion.

The thing is, though, everybody worships. To quote the late David Foster Wallace:

> *The only choice we get is what to worship. And the compelling reason for maybe choosing some sort of god or spiritual-type thing to worship...is that pretty much anything else you worship will eat you alive. If you worship money and things, if they are where you tap real meaning in life, then you will never have enough.... Worship your body and beauty and sexual allure and you will always feel ugly. And when time and age start showing, you will die a million deaths before they finally grieve you.*[1]

Humans are inherently spiritual. For the entirety of our recorded history, we have called to higher authority, whether that authority is a bearded white man on a chapel ceiling, nameless forces that suffuse the universe, gods who abandon their people until a yellow-haired missionary reintroduces them through a banana stalk, or scientific and philosophical first principles. We appeal to things outside ourselves.

I'm no theologian, and this book is not meant as a theological treatise. I'm not here to tell you which god to worship, which first principles to adopt, or how to use the universe's vibrations to attract the right things into your life. People smarter than me can debate the finer points of scripture, argue the biblical support for Calvin's ideas on atonement, and dissect the soteriological implications of certain Greek words. That's not what I want to do.

Instead, this chapter is deeply personal. I want to talk about the felling of the third pillar of my childhood ethic, and I want to tell you what grew in its place. I want to talk about how solving for why has been inextricably linked to worship in my own story.

THROUGHOUT THIS BOOK, MENTIONS of my faith haven't been altogether salutary. That's because, until recently, I couldn't reconcile the faith of my youth with my values, a fact that would eventually force me to abandon one or the other. And nothing is scarier than losing your faith—especially when that's what your faith has taught you.

I grew up under two flinty, absolutist traditions: Catholicism and the American Evangelical church. The *Catechism of the Catholic Church* heralds its absolutism like a town crier: "Outside the Church," it reads, "there is no salvation."[2]

That's it. Not a lot of nuance; outside of the walls of the Mother Church, there's literal hell to pay. One group is exempt, however: those who haven't heard the Gospel. For them, the catechism says their "invincible ignorance" may open the doors to eternal life.

To bring all people into her fold, the Catholic Church encourages mission work. By preaching the Gospel to the world, she hopes to lead the world to the salvation that's within her walls.

This strikes me as a paradox. If being invincibly ignorant of the Church allows the possibility of salvation, then what is the purpose of preaching to the invincibly ignorant? All it can do is condemn the ones who decide not to sign up—ones who would have been saved otherwise.

There are only two ways I could see this missionary paradox making sense: either the missionary truly believes that *all* truth, the fullness of truth, the fullness of life itself resides within the dogmas of the Catholic Church, or the missionary impulse is a poorly masked crusade to concentrate power and to exclude those on the outside. As a Catholic, I was certain it was the former. Today, I see it as another expression of the ethos of the Other.

Enter Evangelical Protestants, and their own claims on salvation.*

Evangelicals believe in a one-time conversion. At the core of Evangelical theology is the idea that we all must be "born again" (a phrase used only three times in the Bible, two of

---

* The word *Evangelical* is fraught. Christians of all stripes, including Catholics, describe themselves as small-*e* "evangelical," a word that stems from the Greek for "good news." To trace the *e*'s path from lowercase to uppercase is to detail a byzantine (and Byzantine) history of Reformation, philosophy, bloodshed, and revival—which I'm not going to do. Instead, when I talk about the American Evangelical theology of my youth, I refer to a specific strand of Protestant Christianity that adheres to what David Bebbington has called "quadrilateral priorities": conversionism, biblicism, crucicentrism, and advocacy. See Bebbington, *Evangelicalism in Modern Britain: A History from the 1730s to the 1980s* (London: Routledge, 1989).

them by Jesus in a single conversation). For many, this conversion happens instantaneously, at the moment we pray the Sinner's Prayer. We acknowledge our essential sinfulness, our powerlessness against sin, and our need for—and submission to—the saving power of the death and resurrection of Jesus.

In the Gospel of John, Jesus says, "I am the way, the truth, and the life. No one comes to the Father except through me."[3] My Evangelical family has interpreted this as "No one comes to the Father except through praying the Sinner's Prayer and accepting me as their personal Lord and Savior."

American Evangelicals are as missional as their Catholic siblings—sometimes more so. They take to heart Jesus's command at the end of the Gospel of Matthew: "Go and make disciples of all nations."[4]

After the dark-haired summer camp preacher introduced me to the wrath of God, this set up a second paradox: Catholics claimed that salvation only came through the Catholic Church. The Evangelical churches I began attending claimed that salvation only came through praying the Sinner's Prayer. In fact, the pastor of my first Evangelical home spoke often of the specific damnation awaiting Catholics.

Both couldn't be right.

From inside, however, both *felt* right. That they did is testament to the sneaky power of the ethos of the Other and the worship of absolutes. An ardent Catholic turned staunch Evangelical, I espoused a paradoxical faith. Catholics claimed an unbroken line, held in place by the Holy Spirit, to Saint Peter himself. They explained away schisms, violence, and centuries of parallel papacies. Evangelicals, on the other hand, claimed that unbroken lines didn't matter, because only the Bible had been authored by the

Almighty. They ignored the lack of original documents and the historical forces underpinning the formation of the canon itself.

THIS PARADOX BECAME MORE than an academic, theological quandary for me once I left the moving sidewalk. As my values drew me toward justice and toward the Other, I had to grapple with the fact that theology has consequences, and, in the case of my formative faiths, those consequences have not necessarily been great.

If questions like "Were you baptized into the Catholic Church?" or "Have you accepted Jesus as your personal Lord and Savior?" confer membership in a heavenly eternity, then these questions—and the doctrines they create—hold a unique power to ostracize and to Other. Which is exactly what they've done: they've constructed not-so-subtle hierarchies and erected structures of dominance* to keep the Other out.

But here's the thing: Jesus spent far more time talking about love, justice, and the poor than he did about doctrine. In his three years in public, the ostracized carpenter who got himself run out of city after city devoted himself—and, in the end, his life—to loving the Other.

When someone asked Jesus to weigh in on the greatest Jewish commandment, he didn't get into theological quarrels about the nature of salvation or the meaning of his impending death. Instead, he said, "Love."

Love the Lord your God with all your heart, soul, mind, and strength. And love your neighbor as yourself. Period. Everything else is secondary.

---

* I'm indebted to Marcus Borg's *The Heart of Christianity* for this phrase.

Is it important that we don't steal? Absolutely. Is it important that we don't commit murder, that we don't get into unjust sexual relationships, that we avoid anger, that we pray? Sure. Jesus preached an entire sermon on a mountain about some of those things.

But are they most important? Emphatically not. I mean, this isn't my opinion. Jesus actually said they weren't. Love God, and love others. Those were the most important commandments.

I KNOW FRIENDS OF mine will read this book, dear friends who will take issue with the flippancy I've used to describe my faith and to describe our shared theology. Some will take it as evidence that I can't be trusted in matters of doctrine, and that, by claiming that Jesus may not have ascribed to either Evangelical or Catholic dogma, I'm somehow renouncing my faith.

And that will sit poorly with them. They'll wonder, did I *really* mean it when I prayed the Sinner's Prayer? Did I ever really believe? Did my infant baptism stick? Was I ever a true Christian? Because if praying the Sinner's Prayer means once-for-all salvation, how could I write these things with such terrifying glibness? I must never have been a true believer.

To these questioning friends, let me only say this: my Christian faith has become an integral part of my why. At the same time, by many of the metrics I learned for how to define a Christian, you may not think I am one.

The road from the dark-haired summer camp preacher, and his declarations of God's white-hot anger, to where I am has been painful, dark, and tortuous. It's made me lose my faith to regain it. It's made me question what it means to be a Christian, what it means to be a person of faith, and what it means to pursue a path of justice.

My childhood had built filigreed, paradoxical, dogmatic cathedrals around a simple altar. Like Gaudí's famous Spanish basilica, they were never finished: I could always add another ornate theological argument to them.

Solving for why has meant tearing down those cathedrals, piece by piece, to find the simple altar at their center. Once off the moving sidewalk, I had to stop believing in the God I'd been taught, the God whose cathedral admitted only people who assented to certain claims. And losing that faith meant losing my foundation. For a very long time.

REDEMPTION OFTEN COMES IN the dark. For me, it also came in a spreadsheet.

In 2016, I embarked on a pilgrimage. Unhappy with the church I'd been attending, I devoted one year to exploring Christianity. I divided that spreadsheet into twelve months and assigned to each month a single denomination. I picked three churches to attend in each denomination, purposely populating that spreadsheet with the denominations from the far right to the far left, from the almost atheist to the high church.

And I discovered that the Christian tent is large, and that no one orthodoxy defines it. Alongside the gilded Catholics worship the dogmatic Evangelicals, the austere Quakers, and the glossolalic Pentecostals. The Trinitarians and the Unitarians both call themselves Christians. Churches that forbid women from making a sound follow the same God as those that call God Mother.

Pilgrimage opened my eyes to something that's been obvious

to anyone outside, but to which I, on the inside, had been blinded: God—thank God—was bigger than doctrine.

As my why crystallized—as my values narrowed on justice, as my heart turned toward the poor, and as my journey drew me closer to the Other—I could no longer brook a doctrine that Othered. My issue wasn't with faith, specifically. It was with the cathedrals I'd built. It wasn't with the altar, but with the dogma I'd surrounded it in.

Fundamentally, my issue was this: I could no longer call orthodox any set of beliefs that led to an exclusion of the Other—sometimes even an embodied hatred of the Other— while it simultaneously spoke words of love. Drawn to outwardly focused churches during that pilgrimage, churches whose primary mission was love of neighbor, I began to gravitate toward an iconoclastic Jesus. Whatever you do to the least of these, the Iconoclast said—to the outcast, the unseen, the Other—you do to me.

And *that* truth finally set me free.

Why do I still call myself a Christian, then? Not because I believe the religion contains exclusive truth. Not because I assent to an infallible set of mutually exclusive intellectual principles. And not because I believe everyone else should either. "You're gonna have to serve somebody,"[5] Bob Dylan wrote, but who that is remains between you and your why.

I'm a Christian because I fundamentally believe in the story of sacrifice and redemption.

I'm a Christian because, while no philosophy can ever be proven true, I find the philosophy that undergirds Christianity uniquely compelling: love God and love your neighbor. Do unto the least of these.

But most of all, I'm a Christian because I love the Jesus that emerges from the gospels. If you want one story from the scriptures that made me finally fall in love, it's in the Gospel of John, chapter eight.*

A woman, caught in adultery. The men around her want to stone her (but, apparently, not the guy she's sleeping with). Crazily, they're within their rights: they're meting out a biblically mandated punishment for adultery.[6] They're on the correct side of orthodoxy. They're quite literally doing what the Bible tells them they should do.

And Jesus still stops them. "Let him who is without sin cast the first stone," he says in the most famous line from this passage. But that's not what I fell in love with. I fell in love with what he says to the woman after he disperses the rabble:

"Who accuses you?" he asks.

She looks around. "No one."

He responds, "Then neither do I. Go and sin no more."

It's so damned beautiful.

Jesus starts by making the orthodox, the literalists, the clean, the righteous, the dogmatic, the—dare I say it—Christians go away. He scatters the people on the inside, the people who surrounded the adulteress, the people who wanted to do to the Other exactly what the Bible told them to do—the people who were *right*.

Then he makes sure she knows she's safe.

Then he tells her she's safe with him too.

Then—and only then—he says, "OK, now live a better life."

---

* I'm aware that the veracity of this passage is questioned and that the earliest extant manuscripts don't include it.

This is grace. This is redemption. This is justice.

This is my why.

In the end, I've learned that I don't care about orthodoxy. I care about redemption. I've learned that I could do without doctrinal certainty if it means I can be love to (and be loved by) those who've been Othered. I'm drawn to stories of sacrifice and death and resurrection and redemption, because those stories ring true.

I'm drawn to the beauty of the world, the beauty of humanity, the beauty of the outcast, the beauty of my gay and polyamorous and divorced and remarried and monogamous and genderfluid friends because we are all the image of God.

Can your why be found in doctrine? Absolutely. But I found mine among the outcast. I finally found Jesus among the Other. I found him in the church that danced amputated, that sang voiceless, and that smiled scarred.

The rest is dross.

Chapter 23

———— ❦ ————

*If you're going to while away the years, it's far bet-
ter to live them with clear goals and fully alive than
in a fog.*

—HARUKI MURAKAMI

SAMBANY IS A RICE farmer from the southern part of Madagascar. Like 60 percent of farmers in his country, Sambany lives a
subsistence lifestyle.[1] His rice paddy produces enough for his
family to survive, and little more.

Sambany also has a tumor growing off the left side of his
face. He's had it for the last thirty years. He's been to ten different hospitals in Madagascar. Only three of them had surgeons,
none of whom would take him to the operating room.

After three decades, the tumor has grown to over sixteen
pounds. It's larger than his head. Veiny, lobulated, and firm,
the fleshy, parasitic burl hangs off his left cheek. By the time
Sambany arrives on the *Africa Mercy* in 2015, he is a cachectic,
anemic, deconditioned shadow.

Gary Parker and his team removed Sambany's tumor when

Mercy Ships was docked in Toamasina, a port city on the wind-
ward side of Madagascar. To travel from his rice farm in the
south to Toamasina, Sambany had to be carried on someone's
back for two days, just to find the nearest road, and then it was
a six-hour drive up the road to get to the ship.

Like many surgical charities, Mercy Ships offers surgery
for free. The operation, the medications, the rehabilitation, the
recovery—all at no cost to Sambany. But, to make that two-
and-a-half-day trip from the south to the east of Madagascar,
Sambany had to sell his rice farm. He shouldered a catastrophic
financial expense to get his "free" medical care. And Sambany's story isn't unique: a person dies of a surgically treatable
condition every two seconds,[2] and nearly half the world's population is at risk of financial catastrophe if they try to get care
for a surgical disease.[3]

THROUGHOUT THIS BOOK, I'VE extolled the virtues of listening,
of taking a learner's posture toward wonder and failure, and of
finding quiet, numinous moments.

Along the way, it pays to listen to people's stories as well.
Any picture of Sambany is dominated by his tumor. When I
was still on the moving sidewalk, the only thing I would have
seen when I looked at Sambany was his operative plan. I would
have seen a mass to be removed and a face to be reshaped.

As I started to apply the Gary Parker Rule, Sambany himself began to change. He became more than a tumor. I began
also to see the exhaustion in his jaundiced eyes, began also to
see past the tumor to the human behind it.

Both ways of looking at Sambany are important, but both

are insufficient—because it's not as if Sambany didn't know he had a sixteen-pound tumor suspended off the left side of his face for thirty years. He knew.

And there wasn't anything he could do about it. At last count, Madagascar had fewer than eight surgical providers per million people. Contrast this to the United States, which has six hundred thirty-three surgical providers per million people, or Norway, which has over a thousand. Four out of every five Malagasy people are farther than two hours away from their nearest health center. And 95 percent of the country's population would, like Sambany, be driven into poverty by the costs of surgery.[4]

Sambany's tumor is more than a tumor: it is a symptom of the ethos of the Other, of the fact that only 4 percent of the surgeries that Madagascar needs actually happen. Of the cathedrals of dominance we've constructed to keep ourselves safe from people like Sambany. His tumor is the embodiment of the structured evil that, according to Paul Farmer, is poverty.

Getting to the heart of Sambany's story has become my life's work. I didn't find my why in simply treating tumors like his. I found it when I learned to listen to, diagnose, and treat the deeper, underlying, systematic injustices his tumor represents. Solving for why in global surgery has driven me for a decade and a half now. I don't want it to stop.

I'M ALSO EXTRAORDINARILY PRIVILEGED. My why is a lot of fun. It takes me to crazy places. And through it, I get to add a drop into the ocean of those who, like me, want to save the world. We won't succeed—not in my lifetime, not in this century—but, along the way, we will hopefully make a couple of lives better, change a few systems, and train some others to come after us to carry on the work.

Changing the world, however, isn't the purview only of the minority who get lucky enough to go to medical school, lucky enough to stumble onto a hospital ship, lucky enough to meet Gary Parker, and lucky enough to fall into careers treating patients like Sambany, Alimou, Houefassi, Benedictine, Lamine, and Andrew. It's the purview of anyone living in their why.

The Japanese have a concept called *ikigai*.[5] At the center of a cruciate Venn diagram, each person's ikigai is the thing we find at the intersection of four questions: "What am I good at?" "What do I love?" "What does the world need?" and, finally, "What can I be paid for?"

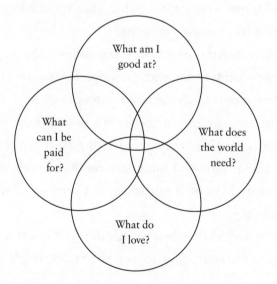

A life that doesn't incorporate all four leads to stagnation. I know. I tried. For nearly two decades, I attempted to be satisfied with three of them: as an academic head and neck surgeon,

I did something I was good at, could be paid for, and, arguably, the world needed more of.* I felt like having three out of the four should have been enough. But I was miserable. I couldn't envisage three more decades of that life. I lived the manila existence of the moving sidewalk: getting by, surviving, and staying safe.

It wasn't until I added the fourth circle in the *ikigai* tetrad that I began to live. Only when I answered, "What do you love?"—and, most importantly, began to pursue it—could I finally stop enduring life until I retired.

YOUR IKIGAI WILL BE unlike mine. Your why is not mine. But if you keep your heart toward the poor, listen to the quiet, numinous moments, find the thin places, face your anxieties, fall in love with failure, and jump off that infernal moving sidewalk, your ikigai can be world changing.

It doesn't matter what your passion is. Do it. Do it to improve the world. In the end, Grandpa Finlay was right: wear out, don't rust out. *In the service of others.*

Solving for why isn't esoteric. It's not limited to those of us who get to work at the coal face of global health. The lessons I've learned are the same lessons that we all learn if we want to create lives of congruence, of purpose, of worth, and of meaning.

And when we do—when we ask the right questions, say yes to the quiet answers, and follow the frustratingly nonlinear

---

* Well, maybe. It's not as bad as Madagascar, but the US suffers under an inequitable distribution of surgeons. Try to convince a hyper-specialized surgeon like me to work in the Ozarks or the Badlands, and you'll be met with ferocious pushback.

path through failures and successes, through contusions and celebrations, through crucifixions and resurrections—we find why.

No matter what you do, keep your eyes on the poor and you can change the world. You *should* change the world. Don't finish your life by meeting the person you could have become. Become that person now.

HERE'S TO YOUR WHY. May you live it well.

Acknowledgments

It may be my name on the spine, but no book is a single person's undertaking. I am deeply indebted to so many people without whom these pages wouldn't have been possible.

My thanks, first of all, to Dana Perino and Erin Landers, who initially put the idea of this book in my head—and who went out of their way to introduce me to folks who would be crucial to its creation. It's no exaggeration to say that this book would never have happened without the two of them.

Many friends and family have slogged through earlier versions of this book. Mia Lazarewicz, Dan Schwarz, Gary Parker, Jay Swanson, Melissa Barre, Ryan Shrime, Souad Shrime, and Peggy Lai, you are all saints for enduring reams of embryonic text. Your guidance has tightened the stories I've told, has corrected me where I strayed, and has encouraged me to keep going during the many nights I just wanted to burn the whole thing down. A special thanks to Mia and to Jay, authors in their own rights, for many all-caps, all-hours text message exchanges about what writing feels like.

The amazing staff at Twelve Books, most especially Rachel Kambury and Sean Desmond, patiently read iterations of this book, maneuvering me through the intricacies of memoir. Thanks also to my agent, Andrew Stuart, and to Liz Segran, who made the initial introduction.

Angelina Krahn's meticulous copyediting has prevented at least six thousand missteps, probably more. Any errors that remain in this book—and I'm sure there are many—are mine alone.

As a surgeon, I've been fortunate to have worked under astonishingly skilled mentors. They are legion, but I'd be remiss not to call out a few in particular: Spiros Manolidis, who first saw surgical potential in me, and who convinced me to consider head and neck cancer surgery as a career; Pat Gullane and Ralph Gilbert, whose technical expertise is surpassed only by the care they have for their patients; and, as always, Gary Parker, who made me the surgeon I am today. I've also gotten to cross paths with surgeons from all over the world, gotten to watch them navigate not only the operating room but also the ministerial and advocacy hurdles necessary to overcome long-ignored barriers to surgical access. They are paragons of perseverance in the service of their patients.

Throughout this weird, convoluted career, I've learned from incredible minds. Joshua Salomon, Milt Weinstein, and Jessica Cohen steadied me through my PhD; John Meara took a chance on me, amplifying my voice in global surgery; and the entire global surgery community have become colleagues and friends since my first post as an academic global surgeon.

The Mercy Ships crew, staff, and volunteers have been nothing but gracious throughout the creation of this book. I particularly want to thank Pauline Rick, Diane Rickard, and Denny Alcorn, who have responded to repeated queries with speed and with grace. And none of this would have been possible had it not been for the vision of Don and Deyon Stephens. Nearly half a century ago, you decided to follow the crazy idea of bringing surgical ships to resource-constrained settings. Your faith has changed many lives, mine included.

To my family: we have been through literal war and death; we have always come out stronger. I pray that never changes.

And finally, to my patients. You are the reason I do what I do. The stories you've told me as I've sat perched on the ends of your beds—stories of strength, of perseverance, of fear, and of faith—have fundamentally changed the way I see the world and my place in it.

Notes

Introduction

1. Valtteri Arstila, "Time Slows Down During Accidents," *Frontiers in Psychology* 3 (2012): 196, https://www.ncbi.nlm.nih.gov/pmc/articles /PMC3384265/.
2. Duan Li et al., "Asphyxia-Activated Corticocardiac Signaling Accelerates Onset of Cardiac Arrest," *Proceedings of the National Academy of Sciences of the United States of America* 112, no. 16 (April 2015): E2073–E2082, https://www.ncbi.nlm.nih.gov/pmc/articles/PMC4413312/.
3. Chess Stetson et al., "Does Time Really Slow Down During a Frightening Event?," *PLoS One* 2, no. 12 (2007): e1295, https://www.ncbi.nlm .nih.gov/pmc/articles/PMC2110887/.

Chapter 1

1. Richard N. Dralonge, ed., *Economics and Geopolitics of the Middle East* (New York: Nova Science Publishers, 2008), 50.
2. Joseph Chamie, "Religious Groups in Lebanon: A Descriptive Investigation," *International Journal of Middle East Studies* 11, no. 2 (April 1980): 175–87.
3. Fawwaz Traboulsi, *A History of Modern Lebanon* (London: Pluto Press, 2012), 91–92.
4. UN General Assembly, Resolution 181 (II), Future Government of Palestine, A/RES/181 (November 29, 1947), https://unispal.un.org/DPA /DPR/unispal.nsf/0/7F0AF2BD897689B785256C330061D253.
5. Benny Morris, *1948: The First Arab-Israeli War* (New Haven, CT: Yale University Press, 2008), 63–79.
6. Telegram from the Department of State to the Embassy in Lebanon, May 19, 1958, 8:57 p.m., document 43, Foreign Relations of the United States, 1958–1960, Lebanon and Jordan, Volume XI, Office of the Historian, US Department of State, https://history.state.gov /historicaldocuments/frus1958-60v11/d43.

7. Dwight D. Eisenhower, Special Message to the Congress on the Situation in the Middle East, January 5, 1957, American Presidency Project, https://www.presidency.ucsb.edu/documents/special-message-the-congress-the-situation-the-middle-east.

8. UPI Archives, "UPI CONTEXT: The Phalange Party of Lebanon," August 29, 1984, accessed Aug. 21, 2020, https://www.upi.com/Archives/1984/08/29/UPI-CONTEXT-The-Phalange-Party-of-Lebanon/6914462600000/.

9. Rola el-Husseini, *Pax Syriana: Elite Politics in Postwar Lebanon* (Syracuse, NY: Syracuse University Press, 2012), 42, 199.

10. Marc Haber et al., "Continuity and Admixture in the Last Five Millennia of Levantine History from Ancient Canaanite and Present-Day Lebanese Genome Sequences," *American Journal of Human Genetics* 101, no. 2 (August 2017): 274–82, https://www.cell.com/ajhg/fulltext/S0002-9297(17)30276-8.

11. Claude Salhani, "Remembering the Lebanese Civil War, 44 Years On," April 4, 2019, *Arab Weekly*, https://thearabweekly.com/remembering-lebanese-civil-war-44-years.

12. George Shrime, typewriter daisy wheel, US Patent 4,714,362, filed June 11, 1982, and issued December 22, 1987.

13. Gary V. Fuller et al., method and apparatus for facsimile enhancement, US Patent 5,224,156, filed July 19, 1990, and issued June 29, 1993.

14. George Shrime, process and means to generate a time indication for different places, European Patent Office, EP0154096A2, filed October 30, 1984.

Chapter 2

1. Erich Bridges, "Tough, Tender Servant to Arab World: Mission Pioneer Finlay Graham Dies," *Baptist Press*, September 8, 2000, accessed August 21, 2020, https://www.baptistpress.com/resource-library/news/tough-tender-servant-to-arab-world-mission-pioneer-finlay-graham-dies/.

Chapter 3

1. Elizabeth Elliot, ed., *The Journals of Jim Elliot* (Revell, 2002), 174.

2. Erin Parke, "The Christian Converts Who Are Setting Fire to Sacred Aboriginal Objects," ABC News Australia, September 19, 2019, accessed August 21, 2020, https://mobile.abc.net.au/news/2019-09-20/the-christian-converts-who-are-setting-fire-to-sacred-aboriginal/11527402; See also Michael Stone, "Pentecostal Christians Are Burning Australia's Sacred Aboriginal Objects," *Progressive Secular Humanist* (blog), *Patheos*, September 19, 2019, accessed August 21, 2020, https://www.patheos.com

/blogs/progressivesecularhumanist/2019/09/pentecostal-christians-are -burning-australias-sacred-aboriginal-objects.

3. Dennis Merritt Jones, *Encouraging Words: Articles & Essays That Prove Who You Are Matters* (Newburyport, MA: Red Wheel/Weiser, 2017), 210.

Chapter 4

1. Paula Span, "A Child's Death Brings 'Trauma That Doesn't Go Away,'" *New York Times*, September 29, 2017, https://www.nytimes .com/2017/09/29/health/children-death-elderly-grief.html.

Chapter 5

1. Center on International Educational Benchmarking, "Singapore: Learning Systems," accessed December 10, 2020, https://ncee.org/what-we-do /center-on-international-education-benchmarking/top-performing -countries/singapore-overview-2/singapore-learning-systems/.

2. Mark Twain, *The Innocents Abroad, or, The New Pilgrims' Progress* (Hartford, CT: American Publishing Company, 1869), 650.

Chapter 6

1. See, for example, Sean Sullivan et al., "Surgical Management of Type II Superior Labrum Anterior Posterior (SLAP) Lesions: A Review of Outcomes and Prognostic Indicators," *The Physician and Sportsmedicine* 47, no. 4 (November 2019): 375–86.

2. Samuel Shem, *The House of God* (New York: Richard Marek, 1978), 390–91.

3. UN Economic Commission for Africa, *The Demographic Profile of African Countries*, March 2016, ix, https://www.uneca.org/sites/default /files/PublicationFiles/demographic_profile_rev_april_25.pdf.

Chapter 8

1. More details on Libby Zion's case can be found at Barron H. Lerner, "A Case That Shook Medicine," *Washington Post*, November 28, 2006, http://www.washingtonpost.com/wp-dyn/content/article/2006/1¼4 /AR2006112400985.html; Steve Cohen, "The Lasting Legacy of a Case That Was 'Lost,'" *Penn State Law Review*, September 28, 2014, http://www .pennstatelawreview.org/penn-statim/the-lasting-legacy -of-a-case-that-was-lost; Dan Collins, "A Father's Grief, a Father's Fight," *Los Angeles Times*, February 1, 1995, https://www.latimes.com /archives/la-xpm-1995-02-01-ls-26834-story.html; "Zion v. New York

Hospital: 1994–95," https://www.encyclopedia.com/law/law-magazines/zion-v-new-york-hospital-1994-95; and Jan Hoffman, "In the Zion Case, a Doctor and Profession on the Stand," *New York Times*, November 19, 1994, https://timesmachine.nytimes.com/timesmachine/1994/11/19/871745.html?pageNumber=27.

2. Nortin M. Hadler, *By the Bedside of the Patient: Lessons for the Twenty-First-Century Physician* (Chapel Hill: University of North Carolina Press, 2016), 80.

3. Sidney Zion, "Doctors Know Best?" *New York Times*, May 13, 1989, https://timesmachine.nytimes.com/timesmachine/1989/05/13/issue.html.

4. "The Public Gains From the Zion Case," editorial, *New York Times*, February 8, 1995, https://timesmachine.nytimes.com/timesmachine/1995/02/08/373495.html?pageNumber=18.

5. Lisa Rosenbaum and Daniela Lamas, "Residents' Duty Hours—Toward an Empirical Narrative," *New England Journal of Medicine* 367, no. 21 (2012): 2044–49.

6. National Residency Matching Program, "2017 NRMP Main Residency Match the Largest Match On Record," March 17, 2017, http://www.nrmp.org/press-release-2017-nrmp-main-residency-match-the-largest-match-on-record/; Association of University Professors of Ophthalmology, *Ophthalmology Residency Match Summary Report 2017*, https://www.sfmatch.org/PDFFilesDisplay/Ophthalmology_Residency_Stats_2017.pdf; "Residents and Fellows," American Board of Dermatology, accessed October 20, 2020, https://www.abderm.org/residents-and-fellows.aspx; "Preventive Medicine Residency Programs," American College of Preventive Medicine, accessed October 20, 2020, http://www.acpm.org/page/pmr.

7. Kaylin Ratner et al., "Depression and Derailment: A Cyclical Model of Mental Illness and Perceived Identity Change," *Clinical Psychological Science* 7, no. 4 (2019): 735–53.

8. Anthony L. Burrow et al., "Derailment: Conceptualization, Measurement, and Adjustment Correlates of Perceived Change in Self and Direction," *Journal of Personality and Social Psychology* 118, no. 3 (2020): 584–601.

9. Kathryn K. Ridout et al., "Physician-Training Stress and Accelerated Cellular Aging," *Biological Psychiatry* 86, no. 9 (2019): 725–30.

10. "Working Hours and Patterns FAQ," NHS Employers, October 12, 2019, accessed August 29, 2020, https://www.nhsemployers.org/pay-pensions-and-reward/medical-staff/doctors-and-dentists-in-training/rostering-and-exception-reporting/working-hours-and-patterns-faqs-updated-august.

11. Asta Medisauskaite et al., "Does Occupational Distress Raise the Risk of Alcohol Use, Binge-Eating, Ill Health and Sleep Problems Among Medical Doctors? A UK Cross-Sectional Study," *BMJ Open* 9, no. 5 (2019): e027362.

12. Anupam B. Jena et al., "Malpractice Risk According to Physician Specialty," *New England Journal of Medicine* (2011): 629–36.

13. Neil Chesanow, "Malpractice: When to Settle a Suit and When to Fight," *Medscape*, September 25, 2013, accessed 29 August 2020, https://www.medscape.com/viewarticle/811323_3.

14. Jonathan Thomas, "The Effect of Medical Malpractice," *Annals of Health Law* 19 (Spring 2010): 306–15.

15. David Hemenway, "Thinking About Quality: An Economic Perspective," *Quality Review Bulletin* 9, no. 11 (1983): 321–27.

16. Robyn S. Shapiro et al., "A Survey of Sued and Nonsued Physicians and Suing Patients," *Archives of Internal Medicine* 149, no. 10 (October 1989): 219–96.

17. Howard B. Beckman et al., "The Doctor-Patient Relationship and Malpractice. Lessons from Plaintiff Depositions," *Archives of Internal Medicine* 154, no. 12 (1994): 1365–70.

18. Charles Vincent et al., "Why Do People Sue Doctors? A Study of Patients and Relatives Taking Legal Action," *Lancet* 343, no. 8913 (1994): 1609–13.

19. Beth Huntington et al., "Communication Gaffes: A Root Cause of Malpractice Claims," *Baylor University Medical Center Proceedings* 16, no. 2 (April 2003): 157–61.

20. Robyn S. Shapiro et al., "A Survey of Sued and Nonsued Physicians and Suing Patients," *Archives of Internal Medicine* 149, no. 10 (October 1989): 219–96.

21. Demetrius Cheeks, "10 Things You Want to Know About Medical Malpractice," *Forbes*, May 16, 2013, accessed August 21, 2020, https://www.forbes.com/sites/learnvest/2013/05/16/10-things-you-want-to-know-about-medical-malpractice/#135e27bc416b.

22. Mark Crane, "Lawsuit: 'The Worst Experience Ever' and 'a Total Surprise,'" *Medscape*, July 23, 2013, https://www.medscape.com/viewarticle/808145.

23. Pauline W. Chen, "When the Doctor Faces a Lawsuit," *Well* (blog), *New York Times*, December 15, 2011, https://well.blogs.nytimes.com/2011/12/15/when-the-doctor-gets-sued-2/.

24. Tait Shanafelt et al., "Burnout and Medical Errors Among American Surgeons," *Annals of Surgery* 251, no. 6 (June 2010): 995–1000.

25. Liselotte N. Dyrbye et al., "Relationship Between Burnout and Professional Conduct and Attitudes Among US Medical Students," *JAMA* 304, no. 11 (2010): 1173–80.

26. Cheryl Clark, "Medical Error 'Second Victims' Get Some Help, Finally," *HealthLeaders*, January 17, 2013, http://www.healthleadersmedia.com /quality/medical-error-second-victims-get-some-help-finally.

27. José R. Guardado, "Medical Professional Liability Insurance Premiums: An Overview of the Market from 2008 to 2017," *Policy Research Perspectives* 2018-2, Economic and Health Policy Research, January 2018, https://www.ama-assn.org/sites/ama-assn.org/files/corp/media-browser /public/government/advocacy/policy-research-perspective-liability -insurance-premiums.pdf.

28. Michelle M. Mello et al., "National Costs of the Medical Liability System," *Health Affairs (Millwood)* 29, no. 9 (September 2010): 1569–77.

Chapter 9

1. Daniel Demesh et al., "The Role of Tonsillectomy in the Treatment of Pediatric Autoimmune Neuropsychiatric Disorders Associated with Streptococcal Infections (PANDAS)," *JAMA Otolaryngology—Head & Neck Surgery* 141, no. 3 (March 2015): 272–75.

2. Mark J. Syms et al., "Incidence of Carcinoma in Incidental Tonsil Asymmetry," *Laryngoscope* 110, no. 11 (November 2000): 1807–10.

3. Colin F. Camerer, (1998). "Prospect Theory in the Wild: Evidence from the Field," *Social Science Working Paper* 1037, Division of the Humanities and Social Sciences, California Institute of Technology, Pasadena, CA, May 1998, https://authors.library.caltech.edu/80314/1/sswp1037.pdf.

4. "2+2=7? Seven Things You May Not Know About Press Ganey Statistics," *Emergency Physicians Monthly*, accessed October 20, 2020, https://epmonthly.com/article/227-seven-things-you-may-not-know -about-press-gainey-statistics/.

5. Morad Chughtai et al., "No Correlation Between Press Ganey Survey Responses and Outcomes in Post–Total Hip Arthroplasty Patients," *Journal of Arthroplasty* 33, no. 3 (March 2018): 783–85; Jessica M. Kohring et al., "Press Ganey Outpatient Medical Practice Survey Scores Do Not Correlate with Patient-Reported Outcomes After Primary Joint Arthroplasty," *Journal of Arthroplasty* 33, no. 8 (August 2018): 2417–22; and Nixon, Devon C. Nixon et al., "Relationship of Press Ganey Satisfaction and PROMIS Function and Pain in Foot and Ankle Patients," *Foot & Ankle International*, July 14, 2020, https://doi .org/10.1177/1071100720937013.

6. E. P. DeLoughery, "Physician Race and Specialty Influence Press Ganey Survey Results," *Netherlands Journal of Medicine* 77, no. 10 (December 2019): 366–69.

7. Lisa J. Rogo-Gupta et al., "Physician Gender Is Associated with Press Ganey Patient Satisfaction Scores in Outpatient Gynecology," *Women's Health Issues* 28, no. 3 (May–June 2018): 281–85.

8. "2+2=7? Seven Things You May Not Know About Press Ganey Statistics," *Emergency Physicians Monthly*, accessed October 20, 2020, https://epmonthly.com/article/227-seven-things-you-may-not-know-about-press-gainey-statistics/.

9. *HCAHPS Stars Ratings Distributions for April 2019 Public Reporting*, Centers for Medicare and Medicaid Services, accessed August 28, 2020, http://www.hcahpsonline.org/globalassets/hcahps/star-ratings/distributions/2019-4-star_ratings_star-distributions.pdf.

10. Shivan J. Mehta, "Patient Satisfaction Reporting and Its Implications for Patient Care," *AMA Journal of Ethics* 17, no. 7 (2015): 616–21.

11. Joshua J. Fenton et al., "The Cost of Satisfaction: A National Study of Patient Satisfaction, Health Care Utilization, Expenditures, and Mortality," *Archives of Internal Medicine* 172, no. 5 (2012): 405–11.

12. Joe Cantlupe, "Expert Forum: The Rise (and Rise) of the Healthcare Administrator," *Athena Health*, November 7, 2017, https://www.athenahealth.com/insight/expert-forum-rise-and-rise-healthcare-administrator.

13. Robert Kocher, "The Downside of Healthcare Job Growth," *Harvard Business Review*, September 13, 2013, https://hbr.org/2013/09/the-downside-of-health-care-job-growth.

14. Christine Sinsky et al., "Allocation of Physician Time in Ambulatory Practice: A Time and Motion Study in 4 Specialties," *Annals of Internal Medicine* 165, no. 11 (December 2016): 753–60.

15. Brian G. Arndt et al., "Tethered to the EHR: Primary Care Physician Workload Assessment Using EHR Event Log Data and Time-Motion Observations," *Annals of Family Medicine* 15, no. 5 (September 2017): 419–26.

16. Danielle Ofri, "The Business of Health Care Depends on Exploiting Doctors and Nurses," *New York Times*, June 8, 2019, https://www.nytimes.com/2019/06/08/opinion/sunday/hospitals-doctors-nurses-burnout.html.

17. Julia E. Szymczak et al., "Reasons Why Physicians and Advanced Practice Clinicians Work While Sick: A Mixed-Methods Analysis," *JAMA Pediatrics* 169, no. 9 (2015): 815–21.

18. Marie Gustafsson Sendén et al., "What Makes Physicians Go to Work While Sick: A Comparative Study of Sickness Presenteeism in Four

European Countries (HOUPE)," *Swiss Medical Weekly* 143 (2013): w13840.

19. Jean E. Wallace, "Mental Health and Stigma in the Medical Profession," *Health* 16, no. 1 (January 2012): 3–18.

20. Tait D. Shanafelt et al., "Changes in Burnout and Satisfaction with Work-Life Balance in Physicians and the General US Working Population Between 2011 and 2014," *Mayo Clinic Proceedings* 90, no. 12 (December 2015): 1600–1613.

21. Louise B. Andrew, "Physician Suicide," *Medscape*, updated August 1, 2018, accessed August 29, 2020, https://emedicine.medscape.com/article/806779 -overview#a.

22. Edward M. Ellison, "Beyond the Economics of Burnout," *Annals of Internal Medicine* 170, no. 11 (June 2019): 807–8.

23. Louise B. Andrew, "Physician Suicide," *Medscape*, updated August 1, 2018, accessed August 29, 2020, https://emedicine.medscape.com /article/806779-overview#a.

24. John C. Goodman, "Why Are Doctors So Unhappy?," *Forbes*, September 14, 2014, https://www.forbes.com/sites/johngoodman/2014/09/11/why -are-doctors-so-unhappy/#44769fe51771.

25. Christina Korownyk et al., "Televised Medical Talk Shows—What They Recommend and the Evidence to Support Their Recommendations: A Prospective Observational Study," *BMJ* 349 (2014): g7346.

Chapter 10

1. Charles Duhigg, "Wealthy, Successful and Miserable," *New York Times Magazine*, February 21, 2019, https://www.nytimes.com/interactive/2019 /02/21/magazine/elite-professionals-jobs-happiness.html.

2. Duhigg, "Wealthy, Successful and Miserable."

3. Sandeep Jauhar, *Doctored: The Disillusionment of an American Physician* (2014; repr., New York: Farrar, Straus and Giroux, 2015), 258.

4. Jim Clifton, "The World's Broken Workplace," *Chairman's Blog*, Gallup, June 13, 2017, https://news.gallup.com/opinion/chairman/212045 /world-broken-workplace.aspx.

5. Susan Adams, "Unhappy Employees Outnumber Happy Ones by Two to One Worldwide," *Forbes*, October 10, 2013, https://www.forbes.com /sites/susanadams/2013/10/10/unhappy-employees-outnumber-happy -ones-by-two-to-one-worldwide/#414f2ed0362a.

6. "Massachusetts Physician Workforce Profile," *AAMC*, accessed August 28, 2020, https://www.aamc.org/system/files/2019-12/state-physician -Massachusetts-2019%5B1%5D.pdf.

7. Shin Ye Kim et al., "Midlife Work and Psychological Well-Being: A Test of the Psychology of Working Theory," *Journal of Career Assessment* 26, no. 3 (August 2018): 413–24.

8. Morten Blekesaune, "Is Cohabitation as Good as Marriage for People's Subjective Well-Being? Longitudinal Evidence on Happiness and Life Satisfaction in the British Household Panel Survey," *Journal of Happiness Studies* 19 (2018): 505–20.

Chapter 11

1. Wayne Brisbane et al., "An Overview of Kidney Stone Imaging Techniques," *Nature Reviews Urology* 13, no. 11 (November 2016): 654–62.

2. John Rawls, *A Theory of Justice* (Cambridge, MA: Harvard University Press, 1971), 11.

3. "Meet the Founder," charity: water, accessed August 28, 2020, https://www.charitywater.org/about/scott-harrison-story.

Chapter 12

1. Maria Cheng, "AP Investigation: Congo Hospitals Openly Jail Poor Patients," *AP News*, October 26, 2018, https://www.apnews.com/86372d0fec5c44bf9760ffa5fe75c2de.

2. "System Performance," *Health Quality Ontario*, accessed August 29, 2020, https://hqontario.ca/System-Performance/Wait-Times-for-Surgeries-and-Procedures/Wait-Times-for-Cancer-Surgeries/Time-to-Patients-First-Cancer-Surgical-Appointment.

3. Aleksandar Hemon, *The Lazarus Project* (2008; repr., New York: Riverhead Books, 2009), 48.

4. Maya Angelou's Facebook page, October 13, 2011, accessed August 28, 2020, https://www.facebook.com/MayaAngelou/posts/10150344661489796.

5. Marcus J. Borg, *The Heart of Christianity: Rediscovering a Life of Faith* (New York: HarperOne, 2009), 133.

Chapter 13

1. I'm indebted for the descriptions of the plight of people with albinism to: UN General Assembly, "Persons with Albinism: Report of the Office of the United Nations High Commissioner for Human Rights," A/HRC/24/57, September 12, 2013, http://www.ohchr.org/EN/HRBodies/HRC/RegularSessions/Session24/Documents/A_HRC_24_57_ENG.doc.

2. Samson Kimaiyo Kiprono et al., "Histological Review of Skin Cancers in African Albinos: A 10-Year Retrospective Review," *BMC Cancer* 14 (2014): 157.

3. Kiprono et al., "Skin Cancers in African Albinos," 157.

4. Mahavagga 11.1, Internet Sacred Text Archive, accessed August 29, 2020, https://www.sacred-texts.com/bud/sbe13/sbe1312.htm.

5. Leo Tolstoy, *A Confession* (Mineola, NY: Dover Publications, 2005), 57.

6. Quoted in *New York Times*, June 20, 1932, 17.

7. Rashid Rashad, *The Power of Family Unity: How to Use It to Gain Economical Freedom for Generations* (self-pub, Xlibris, 2013), 40. Although this quote is often attributed to Mother Teresa, I have been unable to find anywhere she said these exact words. She has, however, expressed similar thoughts, most notably in her Nobel Peace Prize acceptance speech in 1979.

8. "'In the Company of the Poor': Book by Paul Farmer and Fr. Gustavo Gutiérrez," Partners In Health, November 11, 2013, https://www.pih.org/article/in-the-company-of-the-poor.

9. Kwando M. Kinshasa, *Emigration vs. Assimilation: The Debate in the African American Press, 1827–1861* (Jefferson, NC: McFarland & Company, 1988), 128.

10. Maggie Montesinos Sale, *The Slumbering Volcano: American Slave Ship Revolts and the Production of Rebellious Masculinity* (Durham, NC: Duke University Press, 1997), 264.

Chapter 14

1. It's also sometimes called the *optimist criterion*. See Karmen Pažek et al., "Decision Making Under Conditions of Uncertainty in Agriculture," *Poljoprivreda* 15, no. 1 (2009), https://www.researchgate.net/publication/46485867_Decision_making_under_conditions_of_uncertainty_in_agriculture_A_case_study_of_oil_crops.

2. Louis Eeckhoudt et al., *Economic and Financial Decisions Under Risk.* (Princeton, NJ: Princeton University Press, 2005), 3.

3. Pavlo R. Blavatskyy, "Loss Aversion," Working Paper No. 375, Working Paper Series ISSN 1424-0459, Institute for Empirical Research in Economics, University of Zurich, June 2008, http://www.econ.uzh.ch/static/wp_iew/iewwp375.pdf.

Chapter 15

1. Max Deutsch, "M2M Day 243: Attempting to Solve a Saturday New York Times Crossword Puzzle," *Medium*, July 1, 2017, https://medium

.com/@maxdeutsch/m2m-day-243-attempting-to-solve-a-saturday -new-york-times-crossword-puzzle-764b890a216e.

2. Stephen Hiltner, "Will Shortz: A Profile of a Lifelong Puzzle Master," *New York Times*, August 1, 2017, https://www.nytimes.com/2017/08/01 /insider/will-shortz-a-profile-of-a-lifelong-puzzle-master.html.

3. New Year's Resolutions of Americans for 2018, Statista Research Department, *Statista*, accessed August 29, 2020, https://www.statista .com/statistics/378105/new-years-resolution.

4. Rod Sides et al., *2018 Deloitte Holiday Retail Survey: Shopping Cheer Resounds This Year*, 2018, Deloitte Insights, Deloitte LLP, https://www2 .deloitte.com/content/dam/insights/us/articles/4737_2018-holiday -survey/DI_2018-holiday-survey.pdf.

5. Elina E. Helander et al., "Weight Gain over the Holidays in Three Countries," *New England Journal of Medicine* 375 (2016): 1200–1202.

6. Joseph Luciani, "Why 80 Percent of New Year's Resolutions Fail," *U.S. News and World Report*, December 29, 2015, https://health .usnews.com/health-news/blogs/eat-run/articles/2015-12-29/why -80-percent-of-new-years-resolutions-fail.

7. "Mikhail Baryshnikov," *Humanity* (blog), Citizens of Humanity, accessed August 29, 2020, https://mag.citizensofhumanity.com/blog/2015/12/10 /mikhail-baryshnikov.

8. Amos Tversky et al., "Judgment Under Uncertainty: Heuristics and Biases," *Science* 185, no. 4157 (September 1974): 1124–31.

9. Jerome Groopman, *How Doctors Think* (New York, NY: Houghton Mifflin Company, 2008). See also Brent M. McGrath, review of *How Doctors Think*, *Canadian Family Physician* 55, no. 11 (November 2009): 1113.

10. Reshma Saujani, "Teach Girls Bravery, Not Perfection," filmed in Ontario, Canada, February 17, 2016, TED video, 12:31, https://www .ted.com/talks/reshma_saujani_teach_girls_bravery_not_perfection.

11. "Decisions," Doe Zantamata Quotes, accessed August 29, 2020, http://www .doezantamataquotes.com/2013/08/decisions.html.

Chapter 16

1. James Reason, "Human Error: Models and Management," *BMJ* 320, no. 7237 (2000): 768–70.

2. Nathan L. Liang et al., "Outcomes of Interventions for Carotid Blowout Syndrome in Patients with Head and Neck Cancer," *Journal of Vascular Surgery* 63, no. 6 (2016): 1525–30.

3. Brené Brown, *Dare to Lead* (New York: Random House, 2018), 19.

Chapter 17

1. Brené Brown, *Dare To Lead* (New York: Random House, 2018), 19.
2. Dweck's TED talk is worth a listen. Carol Dweck, "The Power of Believing That You Can Improve," filmed at TEDxNorrköping, September 1, 2014, posted November 2014, TED video, 10:13, https://www.ted.com/talks/carol_dweck_the_power_of_believing_that_you_can_improve#t-53420.
3. Merton to Jim Forest, February 21, 1966, in *The Hidden Ground of Love: Letters by Thomas Merton*, ed. William H. Shannon (New York: Farrar, Straus, and Giroux, 1985), 294.
4. Ryder Carroll, *The Bullet Journal Method: Track the Past, Order the Present, Design the Future* (New York: Portfolio/Penguin, 2018), 224.
5. Carol Dweck et al., "A Social-Cognitive Approach to Motivation and Personality," *Psychological Review* 95, no. 2 (1988): 256–73.
6. Bill Hybels, "Leadership Learner," from "Course: 363GLS, Straight from Bill Hybels," Global Leadership Network, accessed August 29, 2020, https://globalleadershipnetwork.org.uk/lesson/leadership-learner/.
7. Quoted in Robert Goldman and Stephen Papson, *Nike Culture: The Sign of the Swoosh* (London: SAGE Publications, 1998), 49.
8. Thich Nhat Hanh and Lilian Cheung, *Savor: Mindful Eating, Mindful Life* (New York: Harper Collins, 2011), 161.

Chapter 18

1. Brendan Murphy, Breaking Down the Numbers Behind the Match Process, *AMA*, January 16, 2018, https://www.ama-assn.org/residents-students/match/breaking-down-numbers-behind-match-process.
2. "9/11 by the Numbers: Death, Destruction, Charity, Salvation, War, Money, Real Estate, Spouses, Babies, and Other September 11 Statistics," *New York*, updated September 2014, accessed August 29, 2020, http://nymag.com/news/articles/wtc/1year/numbers.htm.
3. Electricity Consumers Resource Council (ELCON), "The Economic Impacts of the August 2003 Blackout," February 9, 2004, https://elcon.org/wp-content/uploads/Economic20Impacts20of20August20200320Blackout1.pdf.
4. "Flights Resume, but Situation Remains Tense," CNN, September 14, 2001, http://www.cnn.com/2001/TRAVEL/NEWS/09/13/faa.airports.
5. Ronald C. Kessler et al., "The Epidemiology of Panic Attacks, Panic Disorder, and Agoraphobia in the National Comorbidity Survey Replication," *Archives of General Psychiatry* 63, no. 4 (April 2006): 415–24.

6. "Generalized Anxiety Disorder," National Institute of Mental Health, updated November 2017, accessed August 29, 2020, https://www.nimh.nih.gov/health/statistics/generalized-anxiety-disorder.shtml.

7. Bloomberg, "'We Shouldn't Stop Flying.' What to Make of the Southwest Plane Accident That Shattered a Remarkable U.S. Safety Record," *Fortune*, April 18, 2018, http://fortune.com/2018/04/18/southwest-plane-accident-safety-record.

8. Lydia DePillis, "Lots of Americans Fear Flying. But Not Because of Plane Crashes," *Washington Post*, December 31, 2014, https://www.washingtonpost.com/news/storyline/wp/2014/12/31/lots-of-americans-fear-flying-but-not-because-of-plane-crashes.

9. Charles E. Griffin III et al., "Benzodiazepine Pharmacology and Central Nervous System–Mediated Effects, *Ochsner Journal* 13, no. 2 (Summer 2013): 214–23.

10. Yuka Hayama et al., "The Effects of Deep Breathing on 'Tension-Anxiety' and Fatigue in Cancer Patients Undergoing Adjuvant Chemotherapy," *Complementary Therapies in Clinical Practice* 18, no. 2: 94–98.

11. Katharina Manassis, "Managing Anxiety Related to Anaphylaxis in Childhood: A Systematic Review," *Journal of Allergy (Cairo)* (2012): 316296, https://doi.org/10.1155/2012/316296.

12. Stefan G. Hofmann et al., "The Effect of Mindfulness-Based Therapy on Anxiety and Depression: A Meta-analytic Review," *Journal of Consulting and Clinical Psychology* 78, no. 2 (April 2010): 169–83.

13. Esther M. Blessing et al., "Cannabidiol as a Potential Treatment for Anxiety Disorders," *Neurotherapeutics* 12 (October 2015): 825–36.

14. Michel J. Dugas et al., "A Randomized Clinical Trial of Cognitive-Behavioral Therapy and Applied Relaxation for Adults with Generalized Anxiety Disorder," *Behavior Therapy* 41 no. 1 (March 2010): 46–58.

15. Svein Blomhoff et al., "Randomised Controlled General Practice Trial of Sertraline, Exposure Therapy and Combined Treatment in Generalised Social Phobia," *British Journal of Psychiatry* 179, no. 1 (2001): 23–30.

16. Tone Tangen Haug et al., "Exposure Therapy and Sertraline in Social Phobia: 1-Year Follow-Up of a Randomised Controlled Trial," *British Journal of Psychiatry* 182, no. 4 (2003): 312–18.

17. Fyodor Dostoyevsky, *Winter Notes on Summer Impressions* (1863; repr., Evanston, IL: Northwestern University Press, 1997), 49.

18. Steven C. Hayes, *Get Out of Your Mind & into Your Life: The New Acceptance & Commitment Therapy* (Oakland, CA: New Harbinger Publications, 2005).

19. Lisa Capretto, "Brené Brown on the Two Things Everyone Needs to Live Bravely (Video)," *Huffington Post*, April 23, 2014, https://www .huffpost.com/entry/brene-brown-live-bravely_n_5193927.

20. Marcus Aurelius, *Meditations: A New Translation* (Toronto: Modern Library, 2003), 60.

Chapter 19

1. Kathryn Sketchley-Kaye et al., "Chewing Gum Modifies State Anxiety and Alertness Under Conditions of Social Stress," *Nutritional Neuroscience* 14, no. 6 (November 2011): 237–42.

2. Jim Afremow, *The Champion's Mind: How Great Athletes Think, Train, and Thrive* (New York: Rodale, 2015), 59.

3. Brent S. Rushall et al., "Effects of Thought Content Instructions on Swimming Performance," *Journal of Sports Medicine and Physical Fitness* 29, no. 4 (December 1989): 326–34.

4. Antonis Hatzigeorgiadis et al., "Self-Talk and Sports Performance: A Meta-analysis," *Perspectives on Psychological Science* 6, no. 4 (2011): 348–56.

5. Michael Burgan, *Miracle on Ice: How a Stunning Upset United a Country* (North Mankato, MN: Compass Point Books, 2016), 32.

6. E. M. Swift, "A Reminder of What We Can Be," Vault, *Sports Illustrated*, December 22, 1980, https://www.si.com/vault/1980/12/22/106775781 /a-reminder-of-what-we-can-be.

7. Julie Fuimano, "Staying Positive in a Negative Environment," Biospace .com, September 12, 2006, https://www.biospace.com/article/releases /staying-positive-in-a-negative-environment-/; Daniel Bortz, "Five Ways to Stay Positive During Tough Times,"Monster.com, accessed August 29, 2020, https://www.monster.com/career-advice/article/5-ways-stay-posi tive-in-negativity.

8. Dallas Willard, *Hearing God: Developing a Conversational Relationship with God* (Downers Grove, IL: InterVarsity Press, 2012), 283 (emphasis in the original).

9. Greg Laurie, "Doubt Your Doubts and Believe Your Beliefs," Oneplace .com, accessed August 29, 2020, https://www.oneplace.com/ministries /a-new-beginning/read/articles/doubt-your-doubts-and-believe-your-be liefs-14926.html.

10. David Jeremiah, "How to Battle Against Doubt, Disillusionment, and Discouragement," Crosswalk.com, September 27, 2018, https://www .crosswalk.com/faith/spiritual-life/how-to-battle-against-doubt -disillusionment-and-discouragement.html.

11. Quoted in Wayne Triplett, "Heaven Is Waiting: There's No Place Like Home" (self-pub., iUniverse, 2012), 23 (emphasis mine).
12. Susan David, "The Gift and Power of Emotional Courage," filmed at TEDWomen 2017, New Orleans, LA, November 3, 2017, TED video, 16:40, https://www.ted.com/talks/susan_david_the_gift_and_power_of _emotional_courage.
13. Thomas Merton, *New Seeds of Contemplation* (1949; repr., New York: New Directions, 2007), 12.
14. Angela Lee Duckworth et al., "Deliberate Practice Spells Success: Why Grittier Competitors Triumph at the National Spelling Bee," *Social Psychological and Personality Science* 2, no. 2 (2011): 174–81.
15. Susan David, "The Gift and Power of Emotional Courage," filmed at TEDWomen 2017, New Orleans, LA, November 3, 2017, TED video, https://www.ted.com/talks/susan_david_the_gift_and_power_of _emotional_courage.
16. John Gottman, *Why Marriages Succeed or Fail: And How You Can Make Yours Last* (New York: Simon & Schuster, 1995), 57–58.

Chapter 20

1. M. Giovannini et al., "Gangrenous Stomatitis in a Child with AIDS," *Lancet* 2, no. 8676 (1989): 1400.
2. Joseph E. Tonna et al., "A Case and Review of Noma," *PLoS Neglected Tropical Diseases* 4 no. 12 (2010): e869.

Chapter 21

1. University of Groningen and University of California, Davis, "Average Annual Hours Worked by Persons Engaged for United States," FRED, Federal Reserve Bank of St. Louis, Accessed December 16, 2020, https://fred .stlouisfed.org/series/AVHWPEUSA065NRUG.
2. Larry Page and Sergey Brin, "2004 Founders' IPO Letter: 'An Owner's Manual' for Google's Shareholders," Alphabet Investor Relations, accessed August 29, 2020, https://abc.xyz/investor/founders-letters/2004-ipo-letter.
3. ABA Model Rule 6.1, American Bar Association, accessed August 29, 2020, https://www.americanbar.org/groups/probono_public_service/policy /aba_model_rule_6_1.
4. Jack Kelly, "Finland Prime Minister's Aspirational Goal of a Six-Hour, Four-Day Workweek: Will It Ever Happen?," *Forbes*, January 8, 2020, https://www.forbes.com/sites/jackkelly/202%1/08/finlands-prime -ministers-aspirational-goal-of-a-six-hour-four-day-workweek-will -this-ever-happen/#686801cc3638.

5. David Foster Wallace, "Transcription of the 2005 Kenyon Commencement Address," May 21, 2005, https://web.ics.purdue.edu/~drkelly/DFW KenyonAddress2005.pdf.

6. John Maynard Keynes, *Essays in Persuasion* (New York: W. W. Norton, 1963), 358–73.

7. Jeroen Nawijn et al., "Vacationers Happier, but Most Not Happier After a Holiday," *Applied Research in Quality of Life 5*, no. 1 (March 2010): 35–47.

8. Gretchen Rubin, *The Happiness Project: Or, Why I Spent a Year Trying to Sing in the Morning, Clean My Closets, Fight Right, Read Aristotle, and Generally Have More Fun*, rev. ed. (New York: Harper, 2018).

9. Philippe Tessier et al., "Does the Relationship Between Health-Related Quality of Life and Subjective Well-Being Change over Time? An Exploratory Study Among Breast Cancer Patients," *Social Science & Medicine* 174 (February 2017): 96–103.

10. Philip Brickman and Donald T. Campbell, "Hedonic Relativism and Planning the Good Society," in *Adaptation-Level Theory: A Symposium*, ed. Mortimer H. Appley (New York: Academic Press, 1971), 287–302.

11. National Institute on Drug Abuse, "Cocaine Research Report: How Does Cocaine Produce Its Effects?," May 2016, accessed August 29, 2020, https://www.drugabuse.gov/publications/research-reports/cocaine/how -does-cocaine-produce-its-effects.

12. Edie Weinstein, "Going for the Dopamine High: The Dynamics of Psychopathy," PsychCentral, updated October 25, 2019, accessed August 29, 2020, https://psychcentral.com/lib/going-for-the-dopamine-high-the-dynamics -of-psychopathy/.

13. Swapnil Gupta et al., "Cellular and Molecular Mechanisms of Drug Dependence: An Overview and Update," *Indian Journal of Psychiatry* 49, no. 2 (April–June 2007): 85–90; and Nobue Kitanaka et al., "Alterations in the Levels of Heterotrimeric G Protein Subunits Induced by Psychostimulants, Opiates, Barbiturates, and Ethanol: Implications for Drug Dependence, Tolerance, and Withdrawal," *Synapse* 62, no. 9 (2008): 689–99.

14. Roy F. Baumeister et al., "Some Key Differences Between a Happy Life and a Meaningful Life," *Journal of Positive Psychology* 8, no. 6 (2013): 505–16.

15. Ernest Hemingway, *The Complete Short Stories of Ernest Hemingway: The Finca Vigía Edition* (New York: Scribner, 1987), 275.

Chapter 22

1. David Foster Wallace, "Transcription of the 2005 Kenyon Commencement Address," May 21, 2005, https://web.ics.purdue.edu/~drkelly/DFW KenyonAddress2005.pdf.
2. "Catechism of the Catholic Church," heading for paragraphs 846–48, accessed August 29, 2020, http://www.vatican.va/archive/ENG0015/_P29 .HTM.
3. John 14:6 (CEB).
4. Matthew 28:19 (CEB).
5. Bob Dylan, "Gotta Serve Somebody," track 1 on *Slow Train Coming*, Columbia, 1979.
6. Leviticus 20:10 (CEB).

Chapter 23

1. World Bank Group, *Madagascar Economic Update*, December 2016, https://www.tralac.org/images/docs/10943/madagascar-economic -update-world-bank-december-2016.pdf.
2. John G, Meara et al., "Global Surgery 2030: Evidence and Solutions for Achieving Health, Welfare, and Economic Development," *Lancet* 386, no. 9993 (2015): 569–624.
3. Mark G. Shrime et al., "Catastrophic Expenditure to Pay for Surgery Worldwide: A Modelling Study," in "Global Surgery," special issue, *Lancet Global Health* 3, no. S2 (April 2015): S38–S44.
4. Emily Bruno et al., "An Evaluation of Preparedness, Delivery and Impact of Surgical and Anesthesia Care in Madagascar: A Framework for a National Surgical Plan," *World Journal of Surgery* 41, no. 5 (May 2017): 1218–24.
5. Gordon Mathews, "The Stuff of Dreams, Fading: Ikigai and '"the Japanese Self,'" *Ethos* 24, no. 4 (December 1996): 718–47.

About the Author

Mark G. Shrime, MD, MPH, PhD, FACS, is the O'Brien Chair of Global Surgery at the Royal College of Surgeons in Ireland and a lecturer in the Department of Global Health and Social Medicine at Harvard Medical School.

His academic pursuits focus on surgical delivery in low- and middle-income countries, where he has a specific interest in the intersection of health, impoverishment, and inequity. He is the recipient of numerous awards, including the Arnold P. Gold Humanism in Medicine Award.

When not working, he is an avid photographer and rock climber. He has competed on seasons 8, 9, and 11 of *American Ninja Warrior*. He currently lives in Dublin, Ireland.